The Journey that healed my breasts

Saving Tatas

Christine Austin

BALBOA.
PRESS
A DIVISION OF HAY HOUSE

Balboa Press books may be ordered through booksellers or by contacting:

Balboa Press
A Division of Hay House
1663 Liberty Drive
Bloomington, IN 47403
www.balboapress.com
1 (877) 407-4847

Because of the dynamic nature of the Internet, any web addresses or
links contained in this book may have changed since publication and
may no longer be valid. The views expressed in this work are solely those
of the author and do not necessarily reflect the views of the publisher,
and the publisher hereby disclaims any responsibility for them.

The author of this book does not dispense medical advice or prescribe the use
of any technique as a form of treatment for physical, emotional, or medical
problems without the advice of a physician, either directly or indirectly. The
intent of the author is only to offer information of a general nature to help
you in your quest for emotional and spiritual well-being. In the event you use
any of the information in this book for yourself, which is your constitutional
right, the author and the publisher assume no responsibility for your actions.

Any people depicted in stock imagery provided by Thinkstock are models,
and such images are being used for illustrative purposes only.
Certain stock imagery © Thinkstock.

Print information available on the last page.

ISBN: 978-1-5043-6559-8 (sc)
ISBN: 978-1-5043-6560-4 (hc)
ISBN: 978-1-5043-6593-2 (e)

Library of Congress Control Number: 2016914650

Balboa Press rev. date: 09/10/2016

This book is dedicated to Donna Joanne Herman, my dear mother and closest confidant. After diagnosis in 2005, she endured four surgeries, chemotherapy, radiation, and years of estrogen-blocking hormone medication. She lost the battle on June 3, 2010, ironically, on my father's birthday.

Dear Mother, you are missed more than the sunshine after a long, dreary northeast winter. May you rest in peace, dear one.

If you only knew then what I know now …

ACKNOWLEDGMENT

Special thanks to my dear friend Sarah Munchow for her support and indispensable editing abilities. Good friends are like stars. You don't always see them, but you know they're always there. Thanks for being such a good friend.

CONTENTS

INTRODUCTION

How and why does breast cancer develop? Are random factors merely thrown together, or do they fall neatly into place because of specific genetic and/or environmental factors? How long does the process take? If, indeed, a specific chain of events leads to tumor development, why can't we interrupt the cycle of unhealthy cell production before it becomes untreatable? It is astonishing and ironic that most women still think that breast cancer prevention involves exposing themselves to sensationalized annual breast screenings involving carcinogenic X-rays, simply overlooking entirely the merits of clean eating and environmental chemical exposure.

When I talk to women about breast cancer, I can see the fear in their eyes. They feel helpless to control their breast health and what will become of them as a result. Will they one day find a lump? If and when they do, how will it be evaluated? Will a mammogram find it? Will it have already entered the lymphatic system when detected? Will they lose one or both breasts? Will they have to make life-and-death choices regarding treatment options? Will they have to look someone dear to them in the eye and say those three words: "I have cancer"?

This book is based on my breast cancer scare several years ago. The optional assessment was initiated by me. After my mother's recent diagnosis, I had decided to take some proactive measures to evaluate my breast health, but to be honest, I expected the tatas to be perfectly fine. I was blindsided by the report. It was one of those moments in life when time seems to stand still. There was no past. There was no future. There was only the present moment, and I had to remind myself to breathe. I stared at the words written in black and white laid out before me: "high probability of malignancy." I was about forty years old at the time and still focused on building my career. What a shock. Was I to become a statistic like her?

As you might imagine, after that episode, it was a time in my life filled with fear and angst. Am I really going to follow in my mother's footsteps? What are my viable options? I learned a lot during that time and the weeks to follow. I was blessed to be in the care of a doctor of osteopathy—a DO. She used an approach that is more integrative and proactive. She used techniques, which I will discuss, that most mainstream doctors simply do not recognize or understand. I've tried discussing these groundbreaking methods with mainstream doctors and gynecologists. They tend to look at me like a deer in headlights. They shake their heads and call these methods unproven. But as you will see, they are not unproven, and I am convinced that they can and will save lives. If fact, these methods have likely already saved at least one life—mine.

I looked breast cancer in the face, and I kicked it to the curb. It is possible for many other women and men to do the same. I am confident that if we work together to spread this knowledge, we can hope to virtually eradicate this awful disease. The timeliness is critical. The sooner you receive the assessment, the more time your body has to react to the treatment and heal. I've heard it said that cancer can be in the developmental stages for up to thirty years. That's a lot of time for intervention. Let's not wait until it is too late to take action.

My dear friend Victoria was diagnosed with cancer a few years ago at about age fifty. She chose to have a lumpectomy followed by chemotherapy and radiation. An imaging test called a PET scan was not done after these treatments, perhaps because she told the doctor that she could not afford it. If done, it may have provided an indication as to the effectiveness of the chemotherapy drugs used. Perhaps her treatment could have been more specialized to her. When a PET scan was finally done about two years later, it showed invasive metastasized cancer. She had not been feeling well and feared the cancer had returned with a vengeance. She was right. Her oncologist called to tell her that she was right and he was sorry. The depth of her sadness was extended to her children (my stepchildren) and our grandchildren. You see, the cancer was found too late. Once the cancer has infected the lymph nodes, it spreads quite easily throughout the body. It essentially becomes a death sentence; she was now stage four. Her health continued to decline until December 29, 2014—the day she took her last breath.

The American Cancer Society estimates that one in eight women in the United States, 12 percent, will develop breast cancer during their lifetime. About 232,000 new cases of invasive breast cancer will be diagnosed this year, with 40,000 of those women dying of the disease.[1] No one will be unaffected by breast cancer in some way. Perhaps it will be your mother, wife, or daughter, a co-worker or friend.

According to statistics, women aged between fifty and seventy-four are most at risk of suffering from breast cancer;[2] however, my paternal cousin developed breast cancer in her twenties. The doctors simply ignored her complaints of discomfort, telling her, "You are too young for breast cancer." By the time she was thirty-three, it had invaded her brain and spine. She died leaving three small boys to be raised by a father with no desire nor intention to do so.

I watched my mother go through all facets of the disease. By the time the tumor was discovered by mammogram, it had already invaded the lymphatic system. There were the three surgeries, chemotherapy, radiation, and estrogen blockers—all with their own array of side effects. And it was an illusion that these horrendous treatments could make her well. She continued to struggle with the side effects while watching the calendar for the infamous five-year anniversary. As you will read, she did not make that five-year benchmark. Her life was also taken by this hideous disease—a disease that may be preventable.

What if I told you that there was a magic pill. When this magic pill is taken, you may be able to avert breast cancer, essentially stopping the abnormal proliferation in its tracks. Although I recommend that you discuss this pill with your doctor, it does not require a doctor's prescription. All it requires is a prescription from yourself that deems you worthy of a healthy and happy life.

There currently are diagnostic tests like the mammogram available for the purpose of detecting breast cancer. Unfortunately, mammograms do not always find tumors in time, if at all. Victoria claims that her tumor was the size of a chicken egg and still wasn't detected by mammogram. In addition, it is questionable to me, and at least one doctor I'm aware of, that compressing a tumor tightly between two glass plates is a suitable idea. Did the cancer spread to the lymph nodes before or after the mammogram?

For my mother, my cousin, and my friend Victoria, the mammogram did not detect the cancer in time for effective remedial action. I am not telling you or willing you to stop getting them. In fact, your doctor may fail to treat you if you do not. I am simply suggesting that you consider adding some additional safe screening tools to your tool belt. For many women with dense breasts like me, another screening tool is going to provide much more thorough results and peace of mind.

Life is a constant journey of self-discovery fraught with obstacles; and without the obstacles, frankly, it might just get a bit boring. I would prefer, however, that these obstacles not be life-threatening to myself or those I love. It is imperative that if you are not already a patient advocate that you become one. With wisdom comes power. Armed with useful information and research, you can make your own decisions, and those decisions should be distinct and suitable for you.

What you are reading is based on my experience and my opinion, which resulted from that experience. I am not a doctor. I am a patient and a patient advocate. My intent is to arm you with valuable information, and your job is to determine its personal effectiveness. I hope that you will use the information and share it with others. I am confident that you will find it helpful and that it will give you hope in a future free of breast cancer for you and those you love. Then perhaps you will have the courage to finally live the life you imagined. So go ahead. Step forward into that new life … and be well.

NOTES

_____
_____
_____
_____
_____
_____
_____
_____
_____
_____
_____
_____
_____
_____
_____
_____
_____
_____
_____
_____
_____
_____
_____
_____
_____
_____
_____

Chapter 1

THE MAMMOGRAM

A wise man makes his own decisions; an ignorant man follows the public opinion.

Perhaps you remember the children's fable about the gingerbread man: (Taken from the audio retelling of The Gingerbread Man by Chris Smith for the Story Museum, Oxford.)

> While baking in the oven, the door flies open, and out he pops, excited to be free from the confines of the oven. The old woman tries to stop him, but he gets away as he sings, "Run, run as fast as you can. You can't stop me. I'm the gingerbread man." He comes upon a cat, a dog, and a cow. All give chase and want to eat him, so he continues to run. He then comes upon a fox. The sly fox says, "Let me help you. I'm your friend. I can take you away from all of this. Hop on my tail, and I'll take you across the river." The gingerbread man carefully considers the proposal and

agrees to be escorted safely across the river where the others cannot reach him. As they enter the water, the fox begins to swim, and the gingerbread man has a lovely view. Soon the clever fox convinces him to hop out onto his nose. When the gingerbread man jumps onto the fox's nose, the fox nods his head, flicks the gingerbread man up into the air, opens his mouth, and gobbles him up with his sharp, sharp teeth. When he is done, he laughs and licks his lips.[1]

If the gingerbread man had only known the fox was not to be trusted, he would likely still be running around. So what might this story tell us? Perhaps someone's eagerness to help you should not be taken as an excuse for blind trust.

In this chapter, we will discuss the mammogram in detail. We will touch on its evolution, intent, and impact on women's health. Is it serving its intended purpose or, like the sly fox, simply selling a false idea? We will discuss a few of the latest research studies, its efficacy, and how this information relates to you. How confident are you in its ability to detect a cancerous lump or, for that matter, to detect abnormal tissue before it becomes cancerous? Are you confident enough in your practitioner and the medical establishment to expect a mammogram to save your life? The mainstream medical community considers doing a mammogram prudent, but trusting in it exclusively may be questionable. Does breast density impact the efficacy of the mammogram and its ability to detect abnormalities? How, then, have women been impacted by the recommendation for this form of breast cancer screening?

If you look up the term *breast cancer* at Wikipedia.org, you will find that breast cancer has been around for a very long time. Discovered in Egypt as early as the sixth dynasty (more than four thousand years ago), the writings describe it as untreatable.[2] The seventeenth-century Greeks thought it generally was caused by imbalances in the fundamental fluids that controlled the body.[3] In the eighteenth century, a wide variety of medical explanations were proposed, including a lack of sexual activity, too much sexual activity, physical injuries to the breast, curdled breast milk, and various forms of lymphatic blockages, either internal or due to restrictive clothing.[4] The nineteenth century wasn't much better; Scottish surgeon John Rodman said that fear of cancer caused cancer, and this anxiety, learned by example from the mother, accounted for breast cancer's tendency to run in families.[5] Throughout the many thousands of years of documented breast cancer, no cure has ever been found.

What Is Mammography?

A mammogram is an X-ray that allows a qualified specialist to examine the breast tissue for anomalies. The breast is squeezed tightly between two glass plates to flatten and spread the tissue, producing a readable image. A screening mammogram is used to look for breast disease in women with no symptoms, while a more thorough diagnostic mammogram is generally used to diagnose breast disease in women who have abnormal symptoms or those who have received an abnormal result on a screening exam. Examples of abnormal conditions might be nipple discharge, pain, and/or a lump. The goal of a screening mammogram is to find breast cancer when it's too small to be felt by a woman or her doctor. To improve a woman's chance for successful treatment and survival, finding cancer early is imperative. A screening mammogram usually takes two X-ray pictures of each breast. Some women, such as those with large breasts, may need to have more pictures to ensure comprehensive analysis.

Diagnostic mammograms, on the other hand, are meant to be a bit more thorough. An abnormal area may be found after reviewing the initial screening views. This first screening might produce a doctor's order for a diagnostic screening to examine the area more closely, which will, unfortunately, expose the woman to more radiation.

A physician who has concerns regarding previous breast issues, including cancer, may also order a diagnostic mammogram. If available, a radiologist may be able to review the images while you are present. In that case, the technician can produce additional images, even magnified views, of problem areas without you having to return for another scheduled appointment. Other types of imaging tests, such as the ultrasound and/or magnetic resonance imaging (MRI), may be considered as an adjunct or replacement to an initial or diagnostic screening, depending on the type of problem and where it is located in the breast.

Cancer.org states the following:

A diagnostic mammogram is usually interpreted in one of three ways:

- It may reveal that an area that looked abnormal on a screening mammogram is actually normal. When this happens, the woman goes back to routine yearly screening.
- It could show that an area of concern *probably is not* cancer, but the radiologist may want to watch the area closely. When this happens it's common to ask the woman to return to be re-checked, usually in 4 to 6 months.
- The results could also suggest that a biopsy is needed to find out if the abnormal area is cancer. If your doctor recommends a biopsy, it does not mean that you have cancer.[6]

In *Short History of Mammography,* Van Steen and Van Tiggelen report that "the first attempts to use radiography for the diagnosis of breast abnormalities were made in the late 1920s, but mammography, as we understand it today, was developed in the 1960s. It took the surgery community more than half a century to accept mammography. From the 60s on, French, Swedish, and North American radiologists made it a well-established technique."[7]

Although the amount of radiation emitted from these screenings has been reduced during the past sixty years, the question remains: Are they safe, and do they contribute in any way to unhealthy breast tissue over time? One of the world's top cancer experts, Dr. Samuel Epstein, states, "The premenopausal breast is highly sensitive to radiation, each 1 rad exposure increasing breast cancer risk by about 1 percent, with a cumulative 10 percent increased risk for each breast over a decade's screening."[8]

With such risk associated with the mammogram, it seems important to ask: How effective are they? In September 2010, the *New England Journal of Medicine*, one of the most prestigious medical journals, published the first study in years to examine the effectiveness of mammograms.[9] It would seem that although helpful to some, they seem to reduce cancer death rates by only 0.4 deaths per one thousand women. So do the benefits outweigh the risks?

Mammogram reports will generally also include an assessment of breast density. The density is generally categorized into one of four groups:

- The breasts are almost entirely fatty.
- There are a few, scattered areas of fibrous and glandular tissue in the breast, making it potentially hard to see small masses.

- The breast has more areas of fibrous and glandular tissue that are found throughout the breast, making it potentially hard to see small masses.
- The breast has a lot of fibrous and glandular tissue. This may make it harder to find a cancer that may be present, as it can blend in with normal tissue.

According to Lusine Yaghjyan and Graham Colditz, "Women with high breast density are four to five times more likely to get breast cancer than women with low breast density."[10]

Mi-Jung Lee of Vancouver never thought she would get breast cancer. She had regular mammograms and lived a healthy lifestyle but found a lump in the spring of 2013. What followed were three surgeries in four months—the last being a mastectomy. She couldn't help but wonder why the mammogram didn't show the cancer, even after a diagnostic screening when she found the lump.[13] What she learned was that dense breast tissue put her at a greater risk of breast cancer because the screening is less sensitive to finding the cancer. In fact, according to Norman Boyd, "Mammography may miss over 1/3 of cancers in dense breasts."[11] It would seem that women who depend on a mammogram to diagnose breast cancer at any stage may be in for an unexpected and potentially lethal surprise. The odds of finding cancer by mammography before it has entered the lymphatic system are not as good as one might be led to believe.

As of this publication, breast density notification laws have been put into effect in twenty-six US states and are pending in nine more. Marijke Vroomen Durning reports the following: "A breast density notification law requires that physicians notify women who have undergone mammography and were found to have dense breast tissue."[12] Dr. Christine Wilson, radiologist and medical director of the screening mammography program of the British Columbia Cancer Agency, says, "If we started to do ultrasounds with everyone with dense breasts, that's quite a burden on the system."[13] The same could have been said at every point in history when a new technology came into practice in the medical field. But best practice today is certainly different from yesterday and will be different tomorrow as we keep learning about the human body. This is exactly why you need to be a patient advocate and push the system to provide the treatment that you deem appropriate to your body and your circumstance. Where you, and all of us, can show a need, progress is possible.

A study printed in *The New England Journal of Medicine* compares the diagnostic performance of digital versus film mammography for breast cancer screening. Table 1 of the study approximates dense breast tissue to be present in 40% of women.[14] Do you know whether your breast tissue is dense? Many women do not. I know that mine are dense, because I was told that at my baseline screening at thirty-eight years old. I am not a bit confident in the notion that a mammogram alone will save me from a stage three breast cancer diagnosis. At the point of mammogram detection, cancer has likely already entered the lymph nodes, creating a potential death sentence. There is a need for the medical establishment to acknowledge better or adjunct tools to evaluate breast tissue, dense or not. To try to prevent false negatives, women might consider "tomosynthesis or 3D mammography which is a newer form of x-ray that claims to significantly reduce patient call-backs. It also increases detection of invasive cancers over traditional digital mammogram."[15] You can discuss this option with your doctor. Keep in mind that as with the 2-D option, you are exposing yourself to radiation. In fact, the newer 3-D procedure has been reported to deliver women twice as much radiation as a standard mammogram.

Also new to breast analysis is the "InveniaT ABUS (Automated Breast Ultrasound System). GE Healthcare, a unit of General Electric Company, introduced the new system in 2013 at the Radiological

Society of North America to address the limitations of the mammography when dense breast tissue is involved. The system is to be used as an adjunct to mammography for screening asymptomatic women with >50% breast density (BI-RADS composition/density 3 or 4). The system features advanced automation features and provides 3D clinical images. Gaining FDA approval in 2014, InveniaTM ABUS has been proven to find 55 percent more invasive cancers after a normal or benign mammographic finding."[16] This pain-free exam takes about fifteen minutes.

My Experience

As I type this, I have a bit of soreness above the nipple of my left breast. A few weeks ago I went to see a gynecologist for my annual exam and cervical Pap smear. My doctor of many years retired a few years ago, and this would be my first meeting with this physician's assistant. I decided upon scheduling to just hurry things along not wait to see the doctor. We had no history together, and after she took the needed Pap culture, she did a breast exam. During the physical exam, she found a large (one-inch) lump at about ten o'clock on the left breast. My breasts, as long as I can remember, have been cystic or lumpy. She mentioned that she had recently found a lump on herself and chose to consult with a surgeon and have it surgically removed. Her lump was nonmalignant. She was concerned and recommended that I follow the same course of action.

The reason I was not concerned was because I know that I have dense, fibrocystic breasts and am familiar with the lumps and locations. I do regular breast exams and know that these cysts fluctuate in size throughout my menstrual cycle and are tender when my caffeine intake is high. She wanted me to get a screening mammogram of the right breast (it had been two years since my last screening) and get a diagnostic mammogram of the left. She advised further that an ultrasound and MRI screening also be done, if needed. Lastly, she wanted to refer me to a surgeon who could remove it.

Many women might have freaked out at this news, but I assure you that I did not. My engineering background not only makes me analytical at times, but it also creates an inclination to question what others might not. I carefully considered the options. I was fairly certain that it was a cyst, and furthermore, if it were a tumor, the last thing that I might want to do is compress it tightly between two glass plates. Unfortunately, that is the first thing that doctors will recommend. On his website (www.mercola.com), Dr. Joseph Mercola, an osteopathic physician and alternative medicine proponent, states, "The Mammogram compresses the breast tightly, which can lead to a dangerous spread of cancerous cells, should they exist."[17]

By the time I reached home, I had made my decision. I would not get a mammogram. I chose as my first course of action, not last as she suggested, to make an appointment with the surgeon. I made this choice not because surgeons like to do surgery, but because I knew he could aspirate it. If no fluid was found, I would consider further testing, with the potential exception of a mammogram.

Before my scheduled appointment, the surgeon's office called my gynecologist and asked for copies of the recent mammogram, which I had not gotten. They then called me to ask if I had followed through with it because they had no record of it. I responded, "No, I have not. I wish to see the surgeon first." Fortunately, even though it may not be standard practice, they complied with my request. I visited the surgeon; he stuck a needle into the lump and extracted more than I thought was possible of an ugly brown fluid. Because cysts, not tumors, contain fluid, I felt quite grateful and pleased by the sight. I thanked him, got up, and went home.

Research

One of the largest and most meticulous studies of mammography ever done, involving ninety thousand women and lasting a quarter-century, has added powerful new doubts about the value of the mammography screening test for women of any age. It found that the death rates from breast cancer and from all causes were the same in women who got mammograms and those who did not. And the screening had harms: One in five cancers found with mammography and treated was not a threat to the woman's health and did not need treatment such as chemotherapy, surgery, or radiation. Not to mention that the screening itself emitted radiation.

The study, published in the *British Medical Journal*, is one of the few rigorous evaluations of mammograms conducted in the modern era of more effective breast cancer treatments. It randomly assigned Canadian women to have regular mammograms and breast exams by trained nurses or to have breast exams alone. This large, twenty-five-year study of Canadian women aged forty to fifty-nine found no benefit for women who were randomly assigned to have mammograms.[18] "It will make women uncomfortable, and they should be uncomfortable," said Dr. Russell P. Harris, a screening expert and professor of medicine at the University of North Carolina, Chapel Hill, who was not involved in the study. "The decision to have a mammogram should not be a slam dunk."[19]

I've heard it said that our immune system is designed to eliminate cancer. According to breast surgeon Susan Love of UCLA, "At least 30 percent of tumors found on mammograms would go away if you did absolutely nothing."[20] In the event that you are diagnosed, perhaps you should consider getting a second opinion, and perhaps even a third and a fourth. See various types of doctors, an MD, an integrative doctor, a functional doctor, and/or a naturopathic physician.

Mammography's benefits have long been debated, but no nation with the exception of Switzerland has suggested the screening be halted. "The Swiss Medical Board, an expert panel established by regional ministers of public health, advised that no new mammography programs be started in that country and that those in existence have a limited, though unspecified, duration. Ten of 26 Swiss cantons, or districts, have regular mammography screening programs. Dr. Peter Juni, clinical epidemiologist at the University of Bern and former member of the Swiss Medical Board, said one concern was that mammography was not reducing the overall death rate from the disease, but increasing over-diagnosis and leading to false positives and needless biopsies."[21]

Mammograms will not *prevent you* from getting breast cancer, and the latest study shows they offer very little benefit in improving your chances of survival if you do have it. Overall, the risks can be shown to outweigh the benefits. So the best strategy, which I encourage all women to embark upon today, is not to simply rely on your yearly mammogram and hope for the best. As we will discuss in later chapters, making lifestyle changes can have a huge impact. Researchers estimate that about 40 percent of US breast cancer cases, or about seventy thousand cases every year, could be prevented by making lifestyle changes.[22] As a patient advocate, consider adding other testing protocols to increase the odds of finding abnormal tissue in time to react to it.

An example of another testing protocol is the thermogram. Here is an image of my first thermology, performed November 7, 2005.

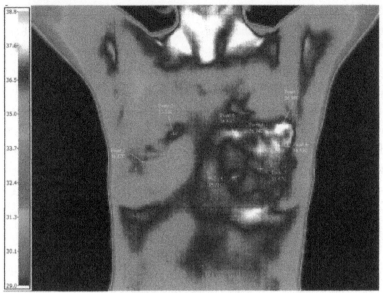

07 November 2005

The use of thermography detected what the mammogram could not. The mammogram, with good intention, did not confirm a lump or abnormal condition neither before nor after the thermogram. The thermal scan, however, shows significant amounts of heat to the right breast, making immediate and proper treatment imperative. If you are thinking, *I wonder what I can do to better my chances of finding abnormal tissue in its early stages of development,* keep reading. We will discuss thermal imaging in more detail in the next chapter.

Notes

Chapter 2

THE THERMOGRAM

You have brains in your head.
You have feet in your shoes.
You can steer yourself,
any direction you choose.
—Dr. Seuss

Early detection is the best prevention.

My Story

It was 2005, and I found myself sitting alone in the doctor's examination room awaiting her appearance. I had withstood the initial cursory review. My vital signs were good, and my weight was, as usual, higher than I deemed appropriate. Feeling a bit anxious, I got up and began to pace about the room.

Due to undiagnosed health issues in my thirties, I had sought out a doctor who was quite thorough and understood the merits of preventive medicine. As I continued to walk about, I noticed some reading material on various conditions and treatments. I picked up a brochure on the thermogram. With my mother's recent breast cancer diagnosis, the information was timely, and it piqued my interest. I was enthralled by the information. I remember thinking, *Why doesn't everyone know about this?* It stated that abnormal tissues could be detected early—before cells become cancerous. This was good news. After all, with regular annual mammograms, my mother's cancer was detected only after it had already spread to the lymph nodes.

After a few questions for the doctor, I decided it would be best to go ahead with the test. Why not? What could it hurt? The test, which at that time cost $100, was not covered by medical insurance. I had just returned to work after twenty-four months of unemployment. Money was tight, but yet, I felt compelled to do something. Taking the test allowed to me feel at least some measure of control over my breast health. Resigning myself to the normal scanning guidelines just didn't feel like enough. I made the appointment and would return to be thermally scanned at a later date.

The option for breast screening that is most highly recommended by well-known author Dr. Mercola is the thermogram.[1] There are no risks, discomfort, or side-effects to using thermograph. There is no discomfort, because a thermogram does not compress tissue; it simply takes a picture. There are no side effects, because it does not expose the patient to radiation.

When you get a thermogram, you will receive a color image. The differing colors on the image represent the differing temperatures of the tissue. The customary mammogram, for example, is devised to check for basic structure. It is looking for a construct or element that should not be there. "By contrast, thermography tests for *physiological change* and *metabolic processes*. It measures the amount of body heat delivered to your skin through cellular metabolism and your nervous system."[2] In other words, inflammation or abnormal tissue will be warmer than the normal, surrounding tissue and will, therefore, show as a different color in this test.

Your external skin temperature can indicate an internal pattern of activity. This preemptive screening can show disturbances in tissue, such as inflammation and/or blockage to the natural lymph flow. These bodily stresses can be found and corrected years before they may even show themselves on traditional screening methods. The thermogram provides opportunity for correction.

"Think of thermography as *preventive medicine*, which can be used to detect, control and even prevent serious illness or disease that otherwise may not be diagnosed until it is *well-advanced*."[3]

The limitations of mammography may be a deal breaker. As in my mother's case, a tumor can be present and growing for several years before detection by traditional methods. Thermography, in contrast, is able to show *visibly* the abnormal formation of blood vessels in much earlier stages of development. In other words, when this abnormal tissue exists, there is a formation of a direct supply of blood to cancer or precancerous cells, which is a necessary step before these cells can grow into tumors of size. This unhealthy formation will be hotter, thereby allowing it to be captured via the infrared camera and then analyzed by a professional technician.

"The Thermogram, essentially, allows you to detect the beginnings of disease sooner, so you're able to take appropriate treatment steps to get your body healing right away."[4] So, in theory, we are finding and correcting abnormal cellular processes before they become fanatic free radicals. You could think of it as similar to a Pap smear. When a Pap comes back with an abnormal report, corrective action can be taken to reverse abnormal cellular changes *before* the patient develops cervical cancer. In that sense, with proper preventive measures and treatment, cervical cancer can be prevented. *The same may now true for breast cancer!* I predict that with the use of thermography in conjunction with a blood test to be discussed later, we can save a lot of tatas and, ultimately, save lives.

We now come to an important point. Neither thermography nor mammography can definitively diagnose breast cancer. They are both diagnostic tests that reveal different aspects of the disease process and allow for further exploration. But unlike the mammogram, the thermogram is painless and does not emit radiation. The patient should abstain from using deodorant and refrain from any practice that would affect skin temperature—like tanning, for example. To start the protocol, the patient removes all upper-body clothing and sits in a comfortable chair, preferably a recliner. She or he will sit with the arms raised overhead for about fifteen minutes, drawing excess heat from the torso. Next, the patient will stand in front of an infrared camera, connected to a computer. Keeping the arms raised, the technician will take a series of pictures. During the process, you may be able to catch a glimpse of the colorful images on the computer screen. Next, the patient, using a nearby sink, will rinse his or her hands under cold water for about thirty seconds. This will draw even more heat from the torso, providing better temperature variation definition. The patient walks back to the target area, and the picture protocol is repeated.

To be quite honest, after leaving the doctor's office, I didn't think much about the test. I liked the thought of being proactive versus reactive but didn't in a million years think that the results would be anything but normal. I simply went back to life as usual.

It was not long before I received a voice mail from my doctor stating that she wanted me to call her back at my soonest convenience. Wasn't that interesting? I did not take this message to be good news.

When I called, she was busy. We played phone tag for a while before she simply left a message for me to call her at home in the evening.

We finally talked, and she told me that she had received my test results, and they were not good. She felt it imperative that we take corrective action immediately. My thermogram results came back stating a high probability of malignancy. My scans were reviewed by a certified clinical thermographer, certified by the American Board of Thermology.

Thermogram images are rated from TH-1 to TH-5, with TH-1 being normal and TH-5 being extremely abnormal. The image will show color variation from blue (cooler) to green to pink to orange/red and to yellow (warmer). I have completed ten scans to date, and my left breast typically will show a higher score. The initial scan was done on November 7, 2005, and showed a right breast score of TH-2 and a left breast score of TH-4. In addition, the blood test, which will be discussed in the next chapter, was very discouraging.

My question to her: "How do we know that I don't already have cancer?"

I quickly followed it up with an ultrasound, physical exam, and MRI. The thermogram report in conjunction with the Estrogen Metabolism Assessment Test (discussed later) allowed for good indication of existing conditions and set the stage for preventive corrective action. That was ten years ago, and with continued corrective measures (discussed later), I remain cancer free with two lovely, original, God-given tatas.

"According to Therma-Scan Reference Library, a score of TH-4, defines an abnormal thermology study that is of probable (definition: more likely than not) risk for breast cancer. This result is not a diagnosis of breast cancer, but rather should be regarded as a specific indication of characteristic blood vessel features and/or that metabolic conditions are present that are consistent with breast cancer. It is possible, but unlikely, that non-cancerous conditions or individual characteristics are the basis for this result, especially on an initial study. Above all, this result means you need to consult with your personal physician and obtain prompt and comprehensive testing for breast cancer. The physician is urged to examine you for a mass or abnormal skin changes and refer you for targeted ultrasound, MRI and/or X-ray mammography, keeping in mind that *a positive thermogram can precede positive results from other objective testing by 5-8 years.* They also recommend a thermology restudy, on a schedule specified in your own report, as an important part of a comprehensive testing panel. Your physician may learn more about breast thermology by visiting the PROFESSIONALS section of the ThermaScan.com website."[5]

My doctor prefers that patients maintain a thermography score at or below TH-3. "The TH-2 score defines a qualified normal result with moderate levels of thermal energy. This score is frequently associated with benign (non-cancerous) conditions such as estrogen-dominant glandular hyperplasia (dense tissue) and fibrocystic disease. The TH-2 score does not indicate breast cancer but it does not rule-out all possibility of breast cancer."[6]

The enactment of the thermogram started a new chapter of life for me. I have no doubt that this scanning protocol, along with another screening tool, provided significant information that when used properly and acted upon, will be shown to extend my life. A former gynecologist once told me that I would be most at risk for a breast cancer diagnosis when I was eleven years younger than my mother's age at diagnosis. With her diagnosis at age sixty-three, that would put my highest risk at age fifty-two, and I'm just about there. With corrective measures that we will discuss later, one of my best scans was in November 2013 when both breasts scored

TH-1. My most recent report states: "Comparative analysis with the 2005 study demonstrates significant decreases in the extent, caliber and relative emission levels of a vascular-like pattern in the cranial aspect of the left breast." Interestingly, improvements took place even with the initiation and continued use of HRT (hormone replacement therapy). HRT will be discussed further in the chapter on supplements.

The thermogram has provided me with peace of mind. Not only do I know where I stand, but I can monitor my progress. The thermogram provides time for repair of an abnormal condition. It establishes a crucial timeline by which corrective measures can be taken before cells become cancerous. How many women after a breast cancer diagnosis wished they could have done something sooner? How many wish they had more time? Of course, I cannot guarantee your results or say whether you will benefit as I have or even if your results will be the same. You can choose to rely, as many women do, on the merits of the mammogram alone, or you can go one step further with the thermogram, quite possibly adding many more years to your life and more life to your years.

Merits

"Initially, thermography was viewed as a competitive tool to mammography, a role for which it was never intended. This is a known fact in the community of board certified clinical thermographers. Thermography is complimentary to mammography and an adjunctive tool in the war on breast cancer. We must learn to accept the information these tools bring to us, and use the information to the best management of the patient, you and me."[7]

If your doctor is not on board with the merits of using thermography, find one who is. You need not give up the mammogram, but using thermography in conjunction with mammography may well save your life. Having a mammogram less often and adding a secondary tool may provide a positive swing in breast health.

According to William Cockburn, DC, "As soon a suspicious (positive) breast thermal examination is performed; the appropriate follow-up diagnostic and clinical testing can be ordered. This could include mammography and other imaging tests, clinical laboratory procedures, nutritional and lifestyle evaluation and training in breast self-examination.

"With this protocol, cancer will be detected at its earliest possible occurrence. It has been estimated by a number of my colleagues that thermography is correct 8-10 years before mammography can detect a mass."[8]

"Thermography is FDA-approved for the detection of breast cancer, when used *in conjunction with mammography*. It does not stand on its own merits. Incidentally, the American Cancer Society does not recommend thermography as a replacement for mammograms. 'Thermography may be used to supplement information from a mammogram and help identify cancers that are close to the skin.' They claim that thermography can't find cancers that are deeper in the breast and it can't detect small cancers."[9]

Thermogram Assessment Services in Palos Verdes, California, in their desire to improve breast cancer survival rates through early detection, recognizes the necessity to assure that thermography exams are performed and analyzed correctly. And in doing so, they claim to be effective at increasing breast cancer survival rates by 61 percent.[10]

So the first image shown here is, again, the first image taken in 2005:

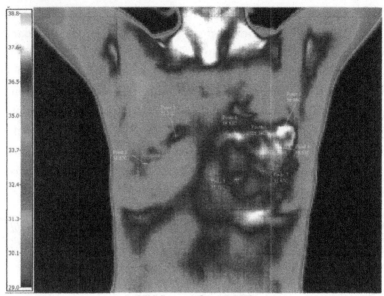

07 November 2005

Now, if you recall, there are surface temperature color variations ranging from blue (29 degrees), green (32.5), pink (35), crimson (36.5), yellow (37.6), and, the warmest, cyan (39). Because these are printed in black-and-white, I will describe the variation: the majority surface temperature is in the pink range. What you see as being very light in color (white) is yellow on the scan, and what appears dark is crimson on the scan. So the right breast appears cool apart from the two crimson locations marked with crosshairs. It scored a TH-2 on the Marseille scoring system, which is the international standard by convention. As we have discussed, the system provides for TH-1 through TH-5 scores as a means of indicating the statistical risk for breast cancer based on the discernment of specific thermology features. The left breast, as you can see, has significantly different surface temperatures, with much of it crimson with spots of even higher yellow temperatures (white here). The left breast scored a TH-4 on the Marseille scoring system.

Now, even though these breast thermology studies are a risk assessment and do not themselves provide a diagnosis of breast cancer, the score of TH-4 merits further evaluation. Due to the score and the report stating there was a high probability of malignancy, I followed up with three screening methods: ultrasound, physical examination, and MRI. I am grateful and happy to tell you that cancer was not found. With that said, action was required to reverse the downward spiral of abnormal tissue development.

The second photo shown here is from January 2016:

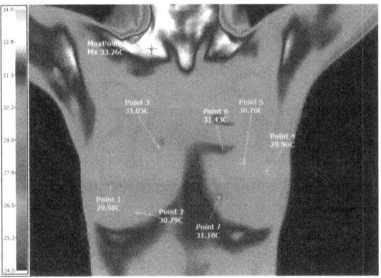

22 January 2016   Front

Even without the benefit of a color image, the improvement in the health of my breast tissue should be apparent. There is no longer any yellow color (white) in the scan, and the crimson color is virtually gone. I would like to thank Therma-Scan Reference Laboratory for the permission to use the images, description, and scoring system.

So how did I heal my tatas? In the next two chapters, I will discuss the methodologies used to facilitate this tissue repair.

NOTES

Chapter 3

ESTROGEN METABOLISM

There is no wealth like knowledge,
and no poverty like ignorance.
—Buddha

It was May 2010, and I was on a business trip in Manhattan. My sister, who lived in our home town, called to tell me about an issue with our mother. It seemed that she had driven herself to the emergency room for treatment, and they were keeping her. She had been complaining about fluid retention and the inability to empty her bladder completely. After an examination, they had scanned her abdomen to find that her liver was full of tumors. Although they never told us, it seemed to have shut down. I called my brothers who lived out of state and told them to come home. It was time to say our good-byes. We did not know it then, but in three weeks, she would be gone forever.

Donna, my mother, was diagnosed with stage three breast cancer in 2005. She had been faithful with her annual mammograms and was therefore surprised when she found the lump. The standard of care would be to have a mammogram, and that is what she did. She *always* had faith and complete trust in her doctors. The mammogram suggested that a biopsy be done. I suspect that a biopsy could have been done without the mammogram; however, doctors tend to follow the designated protocol. With a positive cancer diagnosis, a second surgery was scheduled to check the lymph nodes and take additional tissue for sampling (increase the margins). With most lymph nodes found to be infected, a third surgery was scheduled to take the breast. She wanted the mastectomy with the second surgery, but they would not do it. She was eventually cut vertically from collar bone to belly button. She was prescribed an estrogen-blocking medication and endured radiation and chemotherapy treatments. A fourth surgery placed a chemotherapy port in her chest. It was a difficult journey to say the least, as many of you well know—one that I would not wish on my worst enemy. She did what the doctors asked of her, trusting them with her care and with her life.

Estrogen, a steroid hormone, is present in both men and women. It is found at increased levels in women, most especially in those of reproductive age. Estrogen is known to promote the development of female sexual characteristics and to regulate the menstrual cycle, but as a steroid hormone, estrogen has a wide range of actions and has the ability to affect almost all systems in the body. "In men estrogen regulates certain functions of the reproductive system vital to sperm maturity."[1] "In women, most of the estrogen is produced by the ovaries with smaller amounts produced by the liver, adrenal glands, the breasts, and fat cells."[2] Interestingly, a University of Wisconsin–Madison research team recently reported that even the brain can produce and release estrogen. "Relatively little is known about the control mechanisms of cellular multiplication in normal breast tissue, but evidence seems to indicate that estrogen plays a major role in the development of breast cancer in women and men."[3]

"It is thought that about 80% of breast cancers, once established, rely on supplies of the hormone estrogen to grow. Those cancers are known as hormone-sensitive or hormone-receptor-positive cancers."[4] Therefore, controlling the production of estrogen in the body is a current treatment for these types of cancer. Drugs like Tamoxifen work by blocking the production of estrogen in postmenopausal women. The side effects of these drugs can be so debilitating that some cannot take them. Women can have hot flashes, develop arthritis, and suffer bone loss, thereby affecting their quality of life. Ironically, "Estrogens positively affect the growth, differentiation, and function of various tissues throughout the body—not just those involved in the reproductive process. Estrogens play an important role in bone formation and maintenance, exert cardio protective effects, and influence behavior and mood."[5]

There are three major naturally occurring estrogens in women with a fourth produced only during pregnancy. These major three fluctuate throughout a person's life cycle. Estradiol, the most potent, is the predominant estrogen during reproductive years, while estrone is predominant during menopause. During pregnancy, estriol is the predominant circulating estrogen in terms of serum levels. Like cholesterol, estrogens are not equal.

How Estrogen Is Metabolized

"The metabolism of estrogen takes place primarily in the liver. Some researchers and practitioners now believe that the liver's ability to metabolize estrone is the key to understanding estrogen-related cancer risk. Estradiol is metabolized into estrone, which in turn can be metabolized into either *2-hydroxyestrone or 16-alpha-hydroxyestrone*. While woman have many different estrogens in their body, these estrogen compounds are by far the most important for breast health. 2-hydroxyestrone (2-OHE1) is considered the 'good' estrogen because it does not seem to increase breast cancer risk. This metabolite appears to represent a beneficial direction in estrogen metabolism. The other, 16-hydroxyestrone (16à-OHE1) is considered the 'bad' estrogen because it seems to increase breast cancer risk."[6]

"This metabolite represents a nonbeneficial shift in estrogen metabolism and is associated with a number of problems including lupus, breast cancer, and other estrogen-dependent diseases. All women have both estrogens but at different ratios and more importantly, all women do not metabolize them equally. *Like cholesterol, the ratio is important to breast health.* In general, the higher the ratio, the less association there is with estrogen-dependent diseases. Studies suggest that an Estrogen Metabolism Ratio (EMR) of greater than 0.4 is associated with decreased breast cancer risk in both pre- and post-menopausal women."[7] Are we doing women a huge unnecessary disservice by putting them on an estrogen blocker that blocks all forms of estrogen?

Management of women's health issues with respect to hormones like estrogen is continually changing. I sometimes think that there is no such thing as medical fact, only opinion. In that respect, it is imperative that medical information be scrutinized with an open mind. For example, do you remember when eating eggs were considered harmful because they contain cholesterol? A recent study published in 2013 looked at seventeen prospective studies on egg consumption and health. They discovered that eggs had no association with either heart disease or stroke in otherwise healthy people.[8] In reality, eggs are among the most nutritious foods, containing large amounts of antioxidants lutein and zeaxanthin.

A recent five-year study of 10,786 women was conducted to investigate the role of estrogen metabolism as a predictor of breast cancer, specifically the ratio of 2-OH to 16αOH.[9] The researchers found that "premenopausal women who developed breast cancer had a decreased 2- OH:16α-OH ratio and a higher percentage of 16α-OH than 2-OH. Women with predominately 2- OH were 40% less likely to have developed breast cancer during the 5 years." Another study that began in 1977 found that "premenopausal women who developed breast cancer had a 15% lower ratio than control subjects. Furthermore, those with the highest ratios had about a 30% lower risk to breast cancer than women with lower ratios.[10]"

So it would seem that women who metabolize estrogen into higher levels of 16α-OHE1 may be at higher risk of developing breast cancer. With the ratio of the two being most significant, it would seem that by evaluating a woman's estrogen metabolism, and specifically the ratio of the hydroxylation metabolites, we could predict a woman's breast cancer risk. Furthermore, if we are able to predict high breast cancer risk via analysis of the hydroxylation metabolism, can we follow a protocol to control the ratio, keeping cancer potentially permanently at bay?

It angers and saddens me that this information has been available for some time, and yet, mainstream doctors seem to be unaware of it or are just too busy to wrap their heads around it. I've discussed the estrogen metabolism ratio theory with more than one gynecologist with the same result. They look at me like I am either a crazy b——— or an alien from outer space. In reality, most doctors will simply not use the 2/16 OH Estrogen Metabolism Assessment Test, even though it is widely available and requires only a simple urine or blood sample. This inexpensive technology may have the ability to measure and quantify breast cancer risk long before any actual cancer cells formulate, allowing women to institute corrective measures effectively.

The methods that we will discuss to reverse poor estrogen metabolism do not require a prescription medication. Could it be that the noninvasive technique to hinder cancer development, which I will be discussing, threatens the profits of the mammogram, drug, and surgery cartel that passes for what we consider breast care today? It is my prayer and hope that the breast cancer treatment of tomorrow will be different than the treatment methods of today. It must be. As it is with many ailments, treating the symptoms is just not good enough. We can do better. In reality, women have more control over their breast health than they realize, and *it is time they know it.* With proper education, a woman can have an understanding of the proper care and feeding of her breasts. Armed with useful information, she harnesses the knowledge to circumvent painful surgeries, inhumane chemotherapy, and radiation. Not only that, but we can each play a part in spreading this information.

When I requested the breast thermal scan, my integrative doctor wanted to run this additional test in conjunction with it—this Estrogen Metabolism Assessment Test (Serum). I had never heard of it, but I agreed to have my blood drawn. With my recently learned family history of breast cancer, the more thorough the testing, the better. And if insurance would not cover it, so be it.

It was a few weeks later when I received a call—voice mail, actually—from my doctor, not the nurse, not the medical assistant, but from the doctor herself. The test results were in, and she asked that I return her call immediately. As I discussed in the last chapter, the results were not good, and when combined with the thermal results, my life seemed in jeopardy.

It sounded as though I had caught her at the dinner table, and yet, she was gracious, nonetheless firm. The Estrogen Metabolism Test results were, in her words, "not good." She went on to tell me: "We must take action immediately to reverse this unhealthy metabolic function."

Both of my estrogens were within range; however, my ratio was well outside the recommended healthy range. My ratio was much worse. My bad estrogen was positioned near the right side of the chart, leading to a ratio of about 0.4. By July 2011, I was able to increase the ratio to 0.74.

I have a sister who is three years older than me. A few years ago, I convinced her to also incorporate the breast thermal scan and estrogen metabolism testing into her annual medical protocol. She could not find anyone to provide her the services in her area. Eventually, her only option was to drive the two hundred miles to see my physician. She had the tests done, and the results were equally bad, if not worse. This makes me wonder: Did our mother have the same issue of poor estrogen metabolism? Could she have been saved had she known what I now know? We may never know, but by my sister and me knowing earlier in our lives, we have a great opportunity to do something about it.

What Is Causing Negative Estrogen Metabolism?

If you peruse the Internet, you will find plenty of articles linking estrogen metabolism to breast cancer. Here is a partial list of some of those studies.

Year	Finding
1982	16-alpha-hydroxylated estrogens are associated with breast cancer and suggested to have an etiological role.
1984	Women with breast or endometrial cancer have increased estrogen 16-alpha-hydroxylase activity.
1994	Agents that increase 2-OHE1 inhibit carcinogenesis.

1995	The ratio of 16-alpha OHE1 to 2-OHE1 is elevated in women and animals with high rates of mammary tumors.
1997	Data from women with breast cancer and age-matched controls shows a strong inverse association of the 2/16 ratios with cancer.
2001	2/16 ratio is proposed as a biological marker for risk of head and neck cancer

The big question is this: What causes unbalanced estrogen metabolism, and what can we do about it? Is there a link between our environment as well as what we eat and drink that places us at greater risk? The breast thermal scan report has mentioned pesticides as a possible contributing factor. In later chapters, we will discuss the environment and positive life changes that you can begin to use to increase the odds of living cancer free. We need to find ways to decrease toxins and environmental objects that may be leading to an increase in bad estrogen. In the next chapter, however, we will discuss one corrective measure that can be taken to improve this unhealthy estrogen metabolic state by increasing good estrogen.

In good faith, I should mention that recent research trials have not produced significant or convincing evidence in support of the good versus bad estrogen theory. Again, these studies should be reviewed carefully. For example, what sample size was used? Were the women premenopausal or postmenopausal? Were they on HRT or not? Who did the study? And, perhaps most importantly, who funded the study? I would argue that the proof is in the pudding. In other words, how good is the scientific evidence, and what have you personally experienced? If you searched long and hard, you may find studies that support differing views. A study in 2000, for example, supports the hypothesis that the estrogen metabolism pathway favoring 2-hydroxylation over 16α-hydroxylation is associated with a reduced risk of invasive breast cancer risk in premenopausal women.[11]

I am providing this information because it was crucially important to me with the expectation that it will be valuable to you. My breast health has improved tremendously with treatment and correction of my 2/16 EMR, even while on hormone replacement therapy. In general, clinically positive results have been acknowledged with treatment. In other words, with a change in this ratio, the symptoms of estrogen in the body change. For example, if the ratio of E2 is high or E16 is high and that ratio changes to a better balance of E2, women report less breast pain, fewer hot flashes, easier periods, and cooler thermograms.[12]

NOTES

Chapter 4

SUPPLEMENTATION

> *I'm not lost for I know where*
> *I am. But however, where I am*
> *may be lost.*
> —A.A. Milne, Winnie the Pooh

It was the fall of 2001. I was starting a new volleyball season as coach at the local middle school. There was so much pride and fulfillment in teaching first-year students. Watching them progress from knowing very little about the game to completing a successful season never grew old for me. I loved coaching, but that season was different. I remember sitting my students down on the first night to go over some guidelines for behavior and attendance. As I was speaking, I noticed my vision changing. It was as though a foggy mist was blocking my view, and I struggled to see clearly. I was hot, dizzy, and, it would seem, quite ill. Having a stubborn nature, I pushed through the episodic inconvenience and completed the first lesson. Little did I know that this was the beginning of a downward spiral—one that would last for years.

The constant debility failed to subside, and my symptoms continued to expand. It felt like an infection of some sort. I was so very tired. My body felt heavy, as if I had run a twenty-six-mile marathon twenty-six times. My throat and lymph nodes were sore and swollen. Headaches became quite common. It felt a lot like when I was sixteen years old when and battled the effects of mononucleosis. That was then, but this was now. What was going on? Was it possible that the Epstein-Barr virus was paying me another visit? Weeks went by with no improvement.

I made an appointment with my family physician. It was unfortunate that we did not have much history together. My vital signs were good, and although I felt as if I were running a fever, I was not. I knew that I was very sick. We all have the ability to be keenly aware of our bodies. As individuals, we may know our bodies more intrinsically than any doctor could hope to imagine. I had done my research, and I brought with me a book on chronic fatigue syndrome. I didn't know the cause but was quite certain of my self-diagnosis. To my surprise and dismay, he completely blew me off. He labeled me as tired and sent me home. His apathetic composure was disheartening. I asked for a mono test, and it came back negative. I returned a second time with the same complaints, which led to the same result.

My health continued to decline. By the spring of 2003, I was still employed but taking four naps to get through the workday. It was a constant challenge to even keep my head from bobbing up and down while staring listlessly at my computer. I still do not know the exact cause of my declining health, but I suspect it was a combination of issues. It would seem that I was experiencing some type of endocrine disruptor. After much exhaustion and intense research, I finally found an integrative doctor—out of network and eighty miles from home—who was willing to do some intensive testing. I was found to be deficient in many key nutrients, was toxic with candida, and had high levels of heavy metals in my system. In addition, my endocrine system had basically shut down.

I needed to supplement everything—thyroid, DHEA, adrenals, estrogen, progesterone, thyroid hormone, testosterone, plus key nutrients. I even took IV treatments to jump-start a recovery. It has taken many years to feel human again, and supplements were an essential component in my recovery. My former family physician was quick to prescribe antidepressants and failed, like most physicians, to even consider a root cause. It was a thorough doctor of osteopathy and with the help of nutritional supplements that allowed me to turn a corner.

There is much debate regarding the value of taking vitamin and mineral supplements. Some would claim that by buying and consuming them, you are just creating expensive urine, essentially flushing money down the toilet. If every key essential nutrient were known to man, and you were tested for all of those nutrients and found to be within healthy guidelines, and those guidelines were indeed accurate, the latter statement could be considered accurate.

Let's look at vitamin D, for example. Vitamin D deficiency is extremely common these days and drives a large number of disease processes. There is a growing body of research that clearly shows vitamin D is absolutely critical for good health and disease prevention. Do you know your vitamin D levels? My levels were found to be quite low, and my iodine levels were so low that the data suggested a bodily search for cancer. Your levels of these two key nutrients might play a critical role in an anticancer program.

We may all agree that the most useful and reliable place to acquire nutrients is through the consumption of a healthy diet. Many, however, do not even realize that they are eating unhealthily, and the foods that we have come to believe to be healthy may be tainted with toxic elements like arsenic and/or the herbicide glyphosate. Recent studies suggest that supplementation of certain compounds may play a role in the origin, progression, and therapy for cancer.

Vitamin and mineral products and some food products are currently labeled with a table of recommended daily allowances (RDA). These numbers and percentages are established by the Food and Nutrition Board of the National Academy of Sciences to help the average healthy person maintain good health and avoid nutrient deficiencies. In truth, the allowances succeed in defining the nutrient levels needed to prevent deficiencies that can lead to disease. They seem not, however, to provide sufficient understanding of what nutrient levels promote *optimal* health. There are many factors that can affect how much of any given nutrient is needed by the average person, such as height, weight, genetic factors, and activity level. Which begs the question: Are you average? If you have any intestinal damage due to food allergies, candida, or environmental toxins, for example, the damage that has been done can block nutritional absorption and inhibit proper enzyme production.

This chapter will discuss general nutritional supplementation, as well as a key supplement that may be helpful in the prevention of breast cancer. Recent research data will be helpful in establishing the credibility of responsible vitamin and mineral consumption.

Diindolylmethane

Diindolylmethane (DIM) is both an antioxidant and phytonutrient. It can be found in a variety of cruciferous vegetables, including broccoli, cabbage, and Brussels sprouts, and is formed from the digestion of indole-3-carbinol (I3C). However, in order to get the recommended amount of DIM, one would have to eat at least two pounds of these vegetables daily.

In 1998, University of California, Berkley researchers injected indole-3-carbinol (I3C), a form of DIM, directly into breast cancer cells.[1] The I3C halted the cancer cell division by blocking cancer cell DNA duplication. This led to another study by the same researchers to see if the I3C was as effective as Tamoxifen, which carries numerous undesirable side effects. They injected the first group of human breast cancer cells with I3C, a second with Tamoxifen, and a third with I3C and Tamoxifen. The cells injected with Tamoxifen alone experienced a 60 percent inhibition in DNA synthesis, the cells injected with I3C had a 90 percent inhibition, and the combination had a 95 percent reduction. These studies support the use of I3C for the prevention of recurrence of breast cancer.[2]

There are three basic variations of this type of supplement. There is ample evidence to support the use of DIM, indole-3-carbinol, and/or DIM with calcium D-glucarate for the prevention and treatment of cancer. According to my physician, DIM suppresses bad estrogen, leading to a healthier estrogen metabolism ratio. DIM with calcium D-glucarate (CDG) is recommended in place of DIM for those with a history of cancer. I personally started on DIM with CDG. You can usually find a variation of these supplements at some compounding pharmacies, health food stores, or online; however, my doctor has found the latter version (I3C) to be less effective by mouth than DIM.

"If taken appropriately, DIM is mostly safe, however, taking it in higher than the recommended dose can cause excess gastrointestinal distress and headaches, especially at doses of 300 mg a day and above. Women who are pregnant or lactating should avoid this supplement because there is insufficient safety evidence. People who are at a normal, healthy, weight should consider 100 mg per day. Take 200 mg instead if you are overweight or have significant health concerns because of PMS, menopause, chronic inflammation or a family history of cancers. Always speak with a doctor first as it may interfere with medications."[3] As you monitor your progress via regular blood testing, you will have a better idea of the dosage adequate for your individual needs.

Calcium D-glucarate is a substance made up of calcium and glucaric acid (a chemical compound found naturally in the human body and in a number of fruits and vegetables). Available in dietary supplement form, calcium D-glucarate is said to offer a variety of health benefits, including prevention of cancer.

Although little is known about the safety of long-term use of calcium D-glucarate, there's some concern that taking calcium D-glucarate in combination with certain medications may "decrease the medications' effectiveness. These medications include atorvastatin (Lipitor), lorazepam (Ativan), and acetaminophen (Tylenol) and others. It is always prudent to consult with your doctor before taking any type of supplement."[4]

When seeking to purchase DIM, DIM-CDG, or I3C, you want to feel confident that the supplement will provide meaningful absorption. Buying from a doctor's nutritional pharmacy is one method to achieve that confidence in product quality; another method is to do your research and choose a manufacturer you are comfortable with. A compounding pharmacy is also an option. Keep in mind that if you complete a serum (blood) test to benchmark your estrogen metabolism levels, take a supplement for three months, then retake the test, you should have a good indication of the integrity of the supplement. I recommend this because it provides incentive for continued use.

Keep in mind that some medications are changed and broken down by the liver. It is possible that DIM can have an effect on the breakdown of these medications. Before taking diindolylmethane, talk to your health care provider if you take any medications that are believed to be changed by the liver.[5]

Follow is a list of other supplements to consider after a discussion with your doctor:

Alpha-Lipoic Acid

Discovered in the 1930s, alpha-lipoic acid (ALA) is naturally produced in the body and produced by both plants and animals. "In the late 1980s, scientists realized that alpha-lipoic acid, a compound initially classified as a vitamin when it was discovered, possessed potent antioxidant properties that could prevent healthy cells from getting damaged by unstable oxygen molecules called free radicals. Also known as lipoic acid or thioctic acid, alpha-lipoic acid is mainly derived from dietary sources (spinach, liver, brewer's yeast), although scientists have discovered that the body does manufacture small supplies of its own. In order to get the concentrated doses needed to treat specific ailments, however, many experts recommend supplements."[6]

It can be taken with or without food but is better absorbed on an empty stomach. If you are pregnant, it is always good to discuss supplementation of any kind with your doctor. For supplemental use, ALA holds promise for protecting the body against changes in healthy cells that can lead to cancer. While the body may produce enough lipoic acid, supplementing can allow more optimal levels to circulate readily.

Because lipoic acid works alongside many other nutrients, lack of ALA is difficult to diagnose. "A true deficiency can mimic the general symptoms including weakened immune function, decreased muscle mass and memory problems."[7]

Dosages for ALA can vary by condition. I am currently 600 mg (milligrams) per day to treat high liver enzymes, but for holistic health, I will likely continue to take it. In Europe, 200 to 300 mg a day is frequently used to treat diabetic neuropathy. For use as a general antioxidant, a dosage of 20 to 50 mg daily is often used. Alpha-lipoic acid can be purchased in a variety of dosages. Talk with your doctor about how much alpha-lipoic acid you should take and follow package directions.

Vitamin D

Today's vitamin D (D3) recommendations may be enough to help prevent rickets, but they may do nothing to provide protection from cancer, heart disease, and infections. The recommended dose is 400 to 600 international units (IU) daily; however, most adults may need as much as 8,000 units of vitamin D daily to get blood levels up to healthy levels. It has taken me years to realize my insufficiency and get my vitamin D levels normalized. I find that I need a minimum of 2,000 units daily as a maintenance dose. A blood test will provide the necessary documentation needed by your doctor to recommend your individual daily dosage needs. Keep in mind that vitamin D is one of those nutrients that will not vacate the body naturally. It is fat-soluble and can be taken in excess, so it is best to get tested and follow your doctor's directive regarding dosage.

A PubMed database search found various observational studies regarding the relationship between sufficient vitamin D status and cancer risk. "The evidence suggests that efforts to improve vitamin D status, for example by vitamin D supplementation, could reduce cancer incidence and mortality at low cost, with few or no adverse side effects."[8] Acquiring and taking a vitamin D supplement is not going to break the bank. Despite the hype regarding the dangers of sun exposure, 15 minutes a day can be quite nourishing. There's a reason why our pets tend to lie around in patches of streaming sunlight. In addition, "studies have shown that low vitamin D levels are a risk factor for cancer in general, and particularly for prostate, colorectal, and breast cancers. There are also data that correlate high blood levels of vitamin D with a reduced risk of breast and colorectal cancers. These levels can best be achieved by taking supplemental vitamin D. In colorectal cancer, calcium supplementation may also reduce the risk of polyps (noncancerous growths that may develop on the inner wall of the colon and rectum) and cancer. Numerous studies have tested cancer risk by giving patients supplemental vitamin D, with or without calcium supplementation. While the results are somewhat variable, substantial reduction (on the order of 50%) in the odds of breast and colon cancers with supplementation, have been noted in some studies. Can it stop breast cancer cells from growing? I do not know, but one thing is certain: Vitamin D may play a role in controlling normal breast cell growth. People with a personal history of these types of cancer and their relatives may wish to discuss supplementation with their doctors."[9]

After doing a bit a research, I have no doubt in the efficacy of vitamin D supplementation. "Laboratory studies have shown that vitamin D deficiency can lead to decreased communication between cells and leads them to stop sticking to one another, a condition that could cause cancer cells to spread. Compared with normal cells, cancer cells remain in an immature state, and vitamin D appears to have a role in making cells mature. Vitamin D also appears to play a role in regulating cellular reproduction, which malfunctions (doesn't work properly) in cancer."[10]

Keep in mind, however, that it is possible to take too much vitamin D, perhaps leading to further complications. When you do routine blood work, consider a vitamin D evaluation.

Iodine

Since 1924, iodized salt has been the major source of dietary iodine for Americans. Yet, many of us have been told by the doctor to avoid salt, because salt increases blood pressure. Currently, "15% of the US adult female population is classified by the World Health Organization (WHO) as iodine deficient."[11]

Your breasts contain one of the highest concentrations of iodine in your body, and iodine deficiency is associated with cyst formation. In prolonged iodine deficiency, these nodules become hyperplastic, meaning that an enlargement has formed due to an abnormal multiplication of cells. Hyperplasticity is a precursor to cancer. Thus, long-term iodine deficiency may lead to breast cancer.

According to the late Guy Abraham, MD, our dietary intake of iodine is too low. This was set at 150 mcg (micrograms) per day as the government recommended daily allowance. Dr. Guy Abraham recommended higher iodine intake of 12.5 mg per day, corresponding to the Japanese daily iodine intake. "Higher dietary Iodine may explain why the Japanese have the lowest rates for cancer of the breast, prostate and thyroid."[12]

Dr. B.A. Eskin published eighty papers over thirty years researching iodine and breast cancer, and he reports that iodine deficiency causes breast cancer and thyroid cancer in humans and animals.[13,14] Iodine deficiency is also known to cause a precancerous condition called fibrocystic breast disease.[15] Ghent published a paper in 1993 that showed iodine supplementation works quite well to reverse and resolve fibrocystic changes of the breast, and this is again the subject of a current clinical study.[16,17] You can have your current iodine levels checked via a urine sample. Because my level was shown to be drastically low, I have been taking supplements for several years.

So how much should you take? Stephanie Buist, ND HC, in her guide to iodine supplementation, recommends a maintenance dose up to 50 mg due to more and more exposures to halides bombarding our systems (bromides, fluorides, chlorine), as well as mercury. For cancer patients, an uptick in dosage may be deemed critical. "Cancer is a result of mutated cells. Iodine is absolutely critical for something called P53 gene which is known as the 'keeper of the genetic code.' Without iodine and selenium, it will not function to eliminate abnormal cells from the body such as cancer. Cancer patients have taken anywhere from 50 – 300 mg/day successfully."[18]

Several years ago when I tested and was found to be extremely low in iodine levels, I started on iodine supplementation. In fact, my levels were almost low enough to search the body for cancer. Eventually, I switched to kelp tablets because they are more economical. This might have been a mistake. The kelp tablets contain 150 mcg of iodine, equal to 100 percent of the daily recommended value, but is that enough? After a bit of research, I have realized that I would need to take one hundred of these tablets to improve my iodine levels. 1 mg = 1,000 mcg. Perhaps the higher cost of the higher iodine dosage is worthwhile.

After testing more than five hundred patients, Dr. David Brownstein, a pioneer in the field, found that 94.7 percent of his patients to be deficient in inorganic iodine. David Brownstein said, "After testing individuals and finding low iodine levels, I began to use smaller milligram amounts of iodine/iodide (6.25 mg/day). Upon retesting these individuals 1-2 months later, little progress was made. I therefore began using higher milligram doses (6.25-50 mg) to increase the serum levels of iodine. It was only with these higher doses that I began to see clinical improvement as well as positive changes in the laboratory tests."[19]

Michael B. Schachter says, "The treatment dose when a person is iodine insufficient is generally between 12.5 mg and 50 mg daily. Michael B. Schachter M.D., the medical director of the Schachter Center for Complementary Medicine, is a *magna cum laude* graduate of Columbia College, and received his M.D. degree from Columbia's Physicians & Surgeons in 1965. He is board certified in psychiatry, a certified nutrition specialist, and has achieved advanced proficiency in chelation therapy from the American College for Advancement in Medicine (ACAM). Preliminary research indicates that if a person is iodine insufficient, it takes about three months to become iodine sufficient while ingesting a dosage of 50 mg of iodine and a year to become iodine sufficient while ingesting a dosage of 12.5 mg of iodine daily. However, the patient needs to be monitored closely with awareness of possible side effects and detoxification reactions."[20]

Consult with your doctor to facilitate testing and to discuss proper dosage requirement for optimum health.

Magnesium

"Magnesium is an alkaline earth metal, the eighth most abundant mineral found in the earth's crust. Because of its ready solubility in water, magnesium is the third most abundant mineral in sea water, after sodium and chloride. Unfortunately, it is difficult to reliably supply our bodies with sufficient magnesium, even from a good, balanced whole foods diet."[21] Scholarly articles can be found online that describe how our soils have been depleted of natural magnesium reserves, downgrading the quality of the foods we eat. Both potassium and phosphorus (fertilizers) are adversaries to magnesium in the soil, creating deficiencies at the source. Once food such as fresh produce is picked, handled, transported, stored, and processed, nutrients have already become even more depleted.

"Many partake of a diet of processed, synthetic foods, high sugar content, alcohol and soda drinks that all devastate magnesium levels, as a lot of it is required for the metabolism and detoxification of these largely fake foods. Mental and physical stress, with the continuous flow of adrenaline, uses up magnesium rapidly. If you are supplementing your iron intake, magnesium absorption will be impeded. Many commonly prescribed pharmaceutical drugs cause the body to lose magnesium via the urine, such as diuretics for hypertension; birth control pills; insulin; digitalis; tetracycline and some other antibiotics; and corticosteroids and bronchodilators for asthma. With the loss of magnesium, all of the symptoms being 'treated' by these drugs over time inevitably become worse."[22] It's no wonder there is much current discussion regarding societal magnesium deficiency.

Helayne Waldman, author of *The Whole Food Guide for Breast Cancer Survivors*, claims that "cancer patients generally have a deficiency of magnesium and zinc because that's what people excrete when they're anxious." She recommends replenishing these minerals through supplementation.[23] Whether the cancer or the mineral deficiency comes first, she did not say. Dr. Norm Shealy, one of the world's leading experts on pain and depression management, has found most of his patients to be deficient in magnesium. Many magnesium products are of poor quality and may simply pass through the body, producing a laxative effect. He also notes that patients absorb magnesium much more readily through the skin than by mouth. Dr. Shealy recommends that patients apply two teaspoons of magnesium lotion to the skin twice a day. He sells the lotion on his website, or you can make your own lotion using magnesium flakes purchased from a health food store. Recipes can be found in the next chapter or online.

Kelp also contains magnesium, so you get a double whammy from this supplement—iodine and magnesium. General dosage recommendations for a magnesium supplement by mouth range from about 300 to 400 mg per day, depending upon physical condition and the degree of symptoms. "Oral magnesium supplements are available in organic salt chelates, such as magnesium citrate, and magnesium malate."[22] Other forms include magnesium bicarbonate, magnesium chloride, magnesium hydroxide, magnesium phosphate, magnesium sulfate, and magnesium carbonate obtained from dolomite limestone. Although water-soluble, it may be helpful to divide your dosage throughout the day so that you do not load your body with too much magnesium in any single dose. "Although you may find it helpful for constipation, loose stools indicate you are not absorbing the magnesium, but that it is acting as a laxative. When the magnesium travels through the intestines in less than twelve hours, it is merely excreted rather than absorbed. If you find you cannot overcome the laxative effect by varying your dosages, you may want to try an oral supplement that is chelated to an amino acid, such as magnesium taurate and magnesium glycinate, which some consider to be better absorbed than the salt forms and less likely to cause loose stools."[22]

Another option to supplement your magnesium levels would include a hot Epsom salt bath. Let the water cool a bit while in it for good absorption. Yet another option for oral magnesium supplementation is ionic magnesium in liquid form, such as that offered by Trace Minerals Research. "This is a sodium-reduced concentration of sea water from the Great Salt Lake in Utah. Only about a teaspoon is needed to deliver about 400 milligrams of magnesium (along with seventy-two other trace minerals), which should be taken in divided amounts during the day. Dr. Weston A. Price recommends adding this to soups (made with bone-broth bases of course) as the strong mineral taste is hard to take straight. You can also add this to spring and other drinking water to up the magnesium content and use it in cooking. By 'micro-dosing' your food and water in this fashion you greatly reduce any laxative effects a large dose of magnesium might create."[24]

Zinc

Zinc has been shown to be one of the most important essential trace metals in human health. Zinc is not only a key component in various physiological activities, but when healthy amounts are present in the body via supplementation, it might be considered a drug in the prevention of many diseases. Zinc quickens the activity of many different body enzymes, encourages healthy cell growth and development, fosters immune function to fight illness, and ensures our truc sense of taste and smell.

"An adult's body contains about two to three grams of zinc. It is found in organs, tissues, bones, fluids, and cells."[25] Research by Cardiff University and King's College London in 2012 has identified the switch that releases zinc into cells, with important implications for a number of diseases.

Dr. Kathryn Taylor of Cardiff University's School of Pharmacy and Pharmaceutical Sciences states: "We know that zinc, in the right quantities, is vital for development, our immune systems and many other aspects of human health. But when something goes wrong with the body's zinc delivery system, it looks as though disease can result. In particular, our research has shown a link to highly aggressive forms of breast cancer. Our better understanding of how exactly zinc is delivered suggests if we can block malfunctioning transporter channels, we can potentially halt the growth of these forms of cancer. We believe this makes zinc, and zinc delivery, a high priority for future cancer research."[26]

The recommended daily allowances for men and women are roughly 15 mg and 12 mg, respectively, depending on your source of information. Pregnant women are also at increased risk. Babies in the womb require high amounts of zinc, potentially depleting their mothers of the nutrient. Breast-feeding is another zinc-zapping issue to keep in mind. Be aware that you can get too much of a good thing. Excessive zinc intake can lead to flu-like symptoms, including nausea, diarrhea, vomiting, loss of appetite, abdominal cramps, and headaches. Large doses are used in solid supplements because most of the mineral is thought to be not absorbed. To avoid these side effects, try to keep your zinc intake at or below twice the RDA.

Years ago I had a doctor tell me that white marks on my nails were an indication of zinc deficiency. There is currently controversy regarding this theory, and there are some in the medical establishment who deem the theory to be nothing more than a myth. With that said, I do notice that when I am supplementing daily with zinc, the marks disappear (grow out), and when I stop or take a break, they reappear. I am currently supplementing with ionic zinc sulfate. Nausea can be experienced with zinc supplementation, especially if taken in solid form. The version I take is suspended in de-ionized water, and 1 tablespoon provides 7.5 mg of zinc. The dosage can easily be adjusted if nausea is an issue. My target consumption is 7.5 mg twice a day. I have not experienced any adverse effects from the use of this product.

Vitamin C

Vitamin C is one of those essential nutrients that cannot be made by the body. Instead, it must be attained from the food we eat or the supplements we take. Vitamin C is a water-soluble vitamin and antioxidant, which means that the body uses what it needs and eliminates the rest without dire consequence. Although it may not be sufficient, the recommended dietary allowance of vitamin C for women is about 75 mg per day. Vitamin C supplements are readily available as a powder, in tablets, or as chewable pills at drug stores, most grocery stores, health food stores, and online.

According to Dr. Patrick Holford, "Vitamin C reduces your risk of cancer and high doses are an effective anti-cancer therapy. Of all the antioxidants, vitamin C is the most extraordinary. Vitamin C is believed to help prevent and treat cancer by enhancing the immune system; stimulating the formation of collagen which is necessary for 'walling off' tumors; preventing metastasis (spreading) by inhibiting a particular enzyme and therefore keeping the ground substance around tumors intact; preventing viruses that can cause cancer; correcting a vitamin C deficiency which is often seen in cancer patients; speeding up wound healing in cancer patients after surgery; enhancing the effectiveness of some chemotherapy drugs; reducing the toxicity of some chemotherapy; preventing free radical damage and neutralizing some carcinogens."[27]

The first-ever study in which vitamin C was given to cancer patients was carried out in the 1970s by Dr. Linus Pauling, a biochemist, and Dr. Ewan Cameron, a cancer specialist, working in Scotland. "They gave 100 terminally ill cancer patients 10g (10,000mg) of vitamin C each day and compared their outcome with 1000 cancer patients given conventional therapy. The survival rate was five times higher in those taking vitamin C. By 1978, while all of the 1000 'control patients' had died, 13 of the vitamin C patients were still alive, with 12 apparently free from cancer."[28]

Other studies have confirmed these findings. Dr. Akira Murata and Dr. Fukumi Morishige of Saga University in Japan showed that "cancer patients on 5–30g of vitamin C lived six times longer than those on 4g or less, while those suffering from cancer of the uterus lived 15 times longer on vitamin C therapy."[29] "This was also confirmed by the late Dr. Abram Hoffer in Canada, who found that patients on high doses of vitamin C survived, on average, ten times longer."[27]

However, Pauling and Cameron's findings were discredited, "largely due to an apparent 'replication' of their study by the Mayo Clinic in the US. There was, however, one major difference between the original trial and that of the Mayo Clinic. The 'terminal' patients in the original trial kept taking vitamin C every day, while those in the Mayo Clinic trial stopped after an average of 75 days. However, by then, the book was closed and mega-dose vitamin C was considered quackery."[30] If high doses of vitamin C are thought by anyone to be an effective treatment for cancer, maintaining adequate levels of the nutrient in the body may boost the immune system, thereby allowing protection from the free radicals that can lead to cancer.

There are differing supplementation options, including those with sodium ascorbate, calcium ascorbate, mineral ascorbates, and/or bioflavonoids. There has been some research regarding the various options and whether any one type is better than the other. In one study, "Ester-C® and ascorbic acid produced the same vitamin C plasma concentrations, but Ester-C® produced significantly higher vitamin C concentrations in leukocytes 24 hours after ingestion."[31] Another study, however, found "no difference in plasma vitamin C levels or urinary excretion of vitamin C among three different vitamin C sources: ascorbic acid, Ester-C®, and ascorbic acid with bioflavonoids."[32]

In the United States the recommended dietary allowance for vitamin C was revised in 2000. From the previous recommendation of 60 mg daily for men and women, it was increased to "75 mg for women and 90 mg for men."[33] But keep in mind that these typical RDA values are minimal levels required to prevent chronic disease like scurvy and not necessarily optimum values. It is challenging to find significant data to suggest dosage recommendations of vitamin C for the general prevention of cancer.

I am currently supplementing with a powdered, high-potency buffered vitamin C that is GMO free. One teaspoon mixed with water provides 4,000 mg of vitamin C plus smaller amounts of calcium, magnesium, zinc, and potassium.

Tumeric

A few years ago, I convinced my sister to initiate a more thorough breast assessment. Our mother died of breast cancer in 2010 at the age of sixty-eight. As I have discussed, according to a gynecologist who has since retired, she and I are most at risk eleven years prior to the age at which our mother was diagnosed. With mom diagnosed at sixty-three, my sister is at highest risk at fifty-two. She was about fifty when she was assessed.

She still lives near Toledo, Ohio, where I grew up. We have discussed her challenge to find a physician to provide a thermoscan and estrogen metabolism test. After extensive research, she was forced to invest a few days and drive more than two hundred miles to my clinic in Grand Rapids, Michigan. We are glad that she did. Her results were as bad as mine, if not worse. She was immediately put on I3C. At that time, the clinic did not have the evidence that I3C was not performing as well as DIM for their patients. As previously stated, when I started supplementation, I started on DIM-CDG. This may be why my breast health improved in a few months, while hers has lagged. After a year of supplementation, my sister was not showing much improvement, so they added turmeric with Meriva in the form of a capsule.

Turmeric (Curcuma longa) is dark yellow in color and has been successfully used as powerful medicine in the Chinese and Indian systems of medicine, dating back nearly four thousand years. They use it as an anti-inflammatory agent and antioxidant to treat a wide variety of conditions. The yellow or orange pigment of turmeric is called curcumin. Curcumin is thought to be the primary beneficial agent in turmeric.

As part of the ginger family, it is the root of the plant that we are addressing. The roots are crushed to produce the curcumin extract. It takes roughly twenty pounds of plant root to create two pounds of powdered extract; therefore, a ratio of 10:1 is considered suitable quality. "The oil of turmeric has demonstrated significant anti-inflammatory activity in a variety of experiments."[34] Epidemiological studies have linked the frequent use of turmeric to lower rates of breast, prostate, lung, and colon cancer; laboratory experiments have shown curcumin can prevent tumors from forming; and research conducted at the University of Texas suggests that even when breast cancer is already present, curcumin can help slow the spread of breast cancer cells to the lungs in mice. "Dr. Bharat Aggarwal, Ph.D. Professor, Department of Experimental Therapeutics, Division of Cancer Medicine, The University of Texas MD Anderson Cancer Center, Houston, TX is one of many respected researchers and experts who has published many studies on the effects of curcumin on cancer cells. According to Dr. Aggarwal: 'Curcumin has a very special nature which will work both for cancer prevention as well as for cancer therapy.'"[35]

In one study, published in *Biochemical Pharmacology* (September 2005), human breast cancer cells were injected into mice and the resulting tumors removed to simulate a mastectomy.

> The mice were then divided into four groups. One group received no further treatment and served as a control. A second group was given the cancer drug paclitaxel (Taxol); the third got curcumin, and the fourth was given both Taxol and curcumin. After five weeks, only half the mice in the curcumin-only group and just 22% of those in the curcumin

plus Taxol group had evidence of breast cancer that had spread to the lungs. But 75% of the mice that got Taxol alone and 95% of the control group developed lung tumors.

How did curcumin help? "Curcumin acts against transcription factors, which are like a master switch," said lead researcher, Bharat Aggarwal. "Transcription factors regulate all the genes needed for tumors to form. When we turn them off, we shut down some genes that are involved in the growth and invasion of cancer cells."[36]

In another laboratory study of human non-Hodgkin lymphoma cells published in *Biochemical Pharmacology* (September 2005), "University of Texas researchers showed that curcumin inhibits the activation of NF-kappaB, a regulatory molecule that signals genes to produce a slew of inflammatory molecules (including TNF, COX-2 and IL-6) that promote cancer cell growth. In addition, curcumin was found to suppress cancer cell proliferation and to induce cell cycle arrest and apoptosis (cell suicide) in the lung cancer cells. Clinical trials at the University of Texas are also looking into curcumin's chemo-preventive and therapeutic properties against multiple myeloma and pancreatic cancer, and other research groups are investigating curcumin's ability to prevent oral cancer."[37]

For the most curcumin, be sure to use pure turmeric powder rather than curry powder—"a study analyzing curcumin content in 28 spice products described as turmeric or curry powders found that pure turmeric powder had the highest concentration of curcumin, averaging 3.14% by weight. The curry powder samples, with one exception, contained very small amounts of curcumin."[38]

Turmeric powder should be stored in a tightly sealed container in a dark, cool, and dry place. As with any supplement suggestion, always consult your doctor if you are pregnant or nursing an infant.

Vitamin B6

As we discussed in an earlier chapter, some persons are more likely than others to have dense breast tissue. This dense breast tissue has been shown to challenge the effectiveness of screening. The denser the tissue, the more difficult it can be to detect abnormalities in the breast tissue. The good news is that with my doctor's assistance, I have found a supplement that seems to decrease the soreness and lumpiness that can accompany this anomaly. Whether it helps with screening and detection of abnormal conditions, I cannot say. If you are prone to soreness and or fibrocystic conditions, consider a B6 supplement. I use a time-released formula called Rodex Forte. It is made by a company called Legere Pharmaceuticals in Scottsdale, Arizona. If you cannot procure it online, check with your local compounding pharmacy. If they do not have it, they should be able to order it. I personally find this product to be very helpful.

Hormone Replacement Therapy

At the age of forty-one, I visited my integrative DO for an annual examination and consultation. What took place that day was phenomenal. She rocked my world.

Perimenopause is not for the faint of heart, and unfortunately, with this event, we (women) may bear some of the most uncomfortable side effects known to man. I was experiencing irritability, night sweats, constipation, and more. After some discussion, my doctor wanted to run a serum (blood) test to check my estrogen levels. While we waited for the results to come back, she thought it prudent, based on my symptoms, to go ahead and give me a shot of E-love. I call the estrogen shot E-love because of the dramatic results it provided. It also happened to be my birthday that day. It was the best birthday present a girl could ask for!

Most women can expect to experience perimenopausal symptoms in their forties, but it can start sooner. Not everyone experiences these wildly unpredictable fluctuating hormones in the same way. Some of the most common symptoms are hot flashes that may begin with night sweats prior to menstruation, roller-coaster mood swings, irregular or missed periods, vaginal dryness, low sex drive, short-term memory loss, and insomnia. In short, you might just feel like a crazy woman. Hormone supplementation can ease symptoms; however, studies at the turn of the century revealed a correlation between hormone replacement therapy and an increased risk of breast cancer.

Does Hormone Replacement Therapy Cause Breast Cancer?

In 2012 researchers sought to determine if previous conclusions were correct. "They examined the findings in three studies: the collaborative reanalysis (CR), the Women's Health Initiative (WHI), and the Million Women Study (MWS). In Parts 1–3 of their series of articles the researchers have applied principles of causality to studies analyzing the risk of breast cancer in users of hormone replacement therapy (HRT), as reported from the collaborative reanalysis (CR) (Part 1), and the Women's Health Initiative (WHI) (Parts 2 and 3). In Part 1 they concluded that the CR findings for HRT [both unopposed estrogen therapy (ET) and estrogen plus progestogen (E+P)] did not establish causality. In Part 2 they concluded that the WHI findings for E+P did not establish causality. By contrast, in Part 3 they concluded that valid WHI findings suggested that ET does not increase the risk of breast cancer, and may even decrease it; the latter possibility, however, was statistically borderline. In part 4, they applied causal principles to the evidence from the MWS and concluded that *HRT may or may not increase the risk of breast cancer, but the MWS did not establish that it does.*"[39]

This is a very controversial subject, and there are still many professionals in the health care field who find the risks of use to outweigh the benefits. I might add that to my knowledge, none of these studies used bioidentical hormones versus synthetic.

However, just like many medical opinions, we find the picture of hormone replacement therapy changing yet again, and it is likely to be an ever-evolving conversation. "Cynthia Stuenkel, MD, professor of medicine at the University of California at San Diego says, 'we have had time and resources to carefully tease out the data and perhaps collect a little bit more, and what we have found at least reassures us that for some women who have menopausal symptoms, HRT is not the ominous prescription we thought when the data first came out.' 'We have strong evidence to show that if it is less than 10 years since you started menopause, using HRT on a short-term basis is not likely to harm you, and it can help you; you shouldn't be afraid,' adds Dr. Steven Goldstein, MD, professor of medicine at NYU Medical Center and board member of the North American Menopause Society."[40]

According to Dr. Mercola, alternative medicine proponent, "There are several factors to seriously evaluate when considering if hormone replacement therapy would be wise for you or someone you love:

1. Surgically induced menopause versus natural menopause versus using HRT for preventive purposes.
2. Your age.
3. The form of hormone you take (bioidentical versus synthetic). For example, the WHI study used one specific formulation of HRT called Prempro, which contains potent horse estrogens that are manufactured from the urine of pregnant mares in combination with a synthetic form of progesterone (medroxyprogesterone acetate). It's likely that

bioidentical natural formulations would have resulted in a different outcome.

4.   The manner in which you administer the hormone.

Dr. Mercola suggests that you beware of synthetic hormone usage, as it can cause potential negative side effects. Instead, bioidentical hormones should be considered, because your body recognizes them as normal. There are three types of estrogens commonly used in bioidentical hormone replacement therapy: estrone, estradiol, and estriol. A common mixed formulation known as Tri-est includes 80 percent estriol with 10 percent each of estrone and estradiol. He adds, "It is nearly always wise to use estrogen in conjunction with natural progesterone."[41]

There are a variety of ways that bioidentical hormones may be administered. I used the shot-in-the-hip protocol for about a year to get my levels regulated more quickly. Then I switched over to a patch. Over time, however, I found the patch to be irritating to my skin. I seemed to have a reaction to the adhesive. It was then that I switched to the troche. A troche is mixed at a compounding pharmacy. The liquid is poured into a mold comprising small squares where it will harden as it cools. You simply remove a square per day and place it under your tongue to dissolve. You can choose one of many flavors—I prefer the chocolate myself, which is, incidentally, not a flavor but real chocolate. Bonus!

Another option would be the use of a transdermal cream. However, because hormones are fat-soluble, they can build up in fatty tissues and cause excess amounts in the body. This, consequently, can disrupt other hormones. It's also more challenging to determine the dose accurately when using a cream. Sublingual drops (under the tongue) can be a good option, because it enters your bloodstream directly and will not build up in tissues like the cream may. Required drop dosage may be easier to determine, because one drop is about 1 mg.

An added bonus with compounding your hormones is the ability to accurately prescribe to your needs. In addition, for those with low libido, testosterone can be added to the recipe—another bonus! I am currently taking my estrogen and testosterone in a troche and natural progesterone in capsule form. As we discussed, a troche is a small square that it placed under the tongue to dissolve. All require a prescription and should be thoroughly discussed with your doctor. You should always consider doing your own research online, paying close attention to the parameters of the study or source of information. I have found many studies to be flawed in numerous ways. For example, how many people participated, how old were they, were lumps found before study origination, were synthetic or bioidentical hormones used, and, perhaps most importantly, who funded the study?

I want to take a moment to address my experience with hormone replacement therapy, and this may be the most critical paragraph of this chapter. I received my first thermogram in the fall of 2005, and I started bioidentical HRT in the spring of 2006. Due to my supplementation of DIM, my breast health improved while on the hormone replacement therapy. DIM has also been shown to help with the prevention of abnormal cervical cellular activity. It is now ten years later, and it still has to be the best decision I have ever made, hands down. I have found, for example, when I try to wean off the progesterone, my brain turns to mush and my short-term memory is affected. I would recommend that you become very informed with this topic if you could benefit from HRT and do not let any one mainstream doctor make the decision for you. Always remember that you are the captain of your ship.

NOTES

Chapter 5

GENERAL NUTRITIONAL GUIDELINES

That is the whole secret of successful fighting; get your enemy at a disadvantage.
—George Bernard Shaw

The purpose of food can be defined beyond its ability to stop hunger. Can food be used as medicine? It is becoming more evident that dietary modifications play a critical role in controlling cancer. Anticancer diets are attractive not only for prevention, but for patients who are trying to influence disease progression. According to a major worldwide health organization, up to 30 percent of all cancers might be caused by a poor diet.

In the United States there will be close to three hundred thousand new cases of breast cancer this year, and of those, forty thousand are expected to die of the disease.[1] That's about fifteen deaths for every one hundred thousand cases. The percentage varies and seems to increase with age. In Thailand and Sri Lanka, that number is more in the realm of an astonishing two to five out of one hundred thousand. You could make the argument that the difference in numbers is due to genetic differences, but that seems unlikely since genes are said to influence cancer by approximately 5 percent. In addition, when Asian women move to the United States, they and their daughters suffer an increased risk of breast cancer close to that of American women. When women move from countries with a high breast cancer risk to that of a lower one, their risk declines as well. It is likely environment, diet, and physical activity that protect billions of women in Japan, China, Thailand, Korea, and Africa. Cultural lifestyle seems to play a role along with accessibility to optimum whole foods of high nutrition.

The leading cause of poor eating habits may be misinformation. Fortunately—or, more often, unfortunately—people tend to eat what they are taught to eat. Parental influence on their children creates the very foundation of their belief systems, potentially affecting their decisions for a lifetime. Children tend to have extremely high levels of theta brain waves, which boost their learning ability and provide programming to the subconscious mind. Similar to the hypnotic state, as children we are like sponges absorbing and remembering incredible amounts of information.

Parents have been influenced in a similar manner by their parents, and when combined with their socioeconomic status, these parameters can lead to generations of poor decision-makers. Those of lower socioeconomic status (SES) will find it more difficult to buy high-quality nutrition due to the higher cost and the long-term thought pattern of devaluing the merits of healthy nutrition. This begs the question: Is poverty carcinogenic? Growing up in a lower-middle-class environment, I had no idea how unhealthy I was eating. Common staples were bread, potatoes, meat, and large amounts of junk food. I grew up in the seventies when women were going back to work, and convenient, processed foods were the new fad. Why buy two dollars' worth of greens when you can buy boxes of macaroni and cheese, three for a dollar?

Genetically Modified Organisms (GMO)/Genetically Engineered (GE)/Herbicide Tolerant (GT)

In my childhood home, there were very few fresh fruits or vegetables that I can remember. Canned vegetables were used often at dinner, especially canned corn and green beans. There are some, including myself, who would no longer even consider canned corn a vegetable. Perhaps considered one of the more palatable vegetables by children, the corn of yesterday is not the same as the corn of today, and its nutritional value could be debated. Corn has been labeled by some to be a genetically modified food (GMO) to avoid. According to the US Department of Agriculture (USDA), GMO "corn accounted for 85 percent of corn acreage in 2013. Herbicide-tolerant crops have traits that allow them to tolerate effective herbicides, such as glyphosate, helping to control pervasive weeds more effectively."[2] There is much controversy these days about whether GMO foods are bad for us.

The American Academy of Environmental Medicine (AAEM) has warned that "GMOs pose a serious threat to health. In fact, the AAEM has advised doctors to tell their patients to avoid GMOs. They claim that the introduction of GMOs into the current food supply has correlated with an alarming rise in chronic diseases and food allergies."[3] What you may not realize is that you have been consuming products with GMO ingredients for years. If you peruse the ingredients on a can of soup, for example, you will ultimately find GMO components. In America, says the Non-GMO Project, "90 percent of cottonseed, 90 percent of rapeseed (the source of canola), and 94 percent of soybeans are GMOs."[4]

"The existing few studies that analyzed GM-foods already on the market found that these modified foods were significantly lower in nutritional value than non-GM-foods. This means that the long-term consumption of mainly GM-foods in one's diet could bring about nutritional deficiencies. And when it comes to cancer, nutritional deficiencies have been found to be a major contributing factor."[5] Do your own research to determine if GMO food is right for you.

What you can do: Start to limit or avoid foods that are known to be genetically modified—for example, corn, wheat, and soy. Whenever possible, choose locally grown produce bought directly from the farmer or your local farm market where you can ask questions about production. In addition, nutrients are their highest immediately after picking. Buying locally provides wonderful economic value to the local economy and also provides opportunities for you to learn and acknowledge local growing methods, creating more choice.

Carbohydrates

It is no wonder that many are confused about nutrition. It is an issue that seems to ebb and flow with the tide. Eggs are bad for you. No, no, no … eggs are good for you. Butter, now that is evil. No, no, no … modern margarine with trans fat is what's evil. Butter is now considered fine in moderation. It's enough to make your head spin and supports the notion that one should not always be quick to get on the bandwagon.

Cancer is considered by some to be a modern disease. After switching from a high-protein, high-fat, moderate-carb, low-toxin diet to a grain-based diet, people started getting cancer in greater numbers. "German researchers from the University Hospital of Würzburg published one of the largest reviews on the benefits of low-carbohydrate diets for cancer patients. This study is one of the best showing a high-carb, grain based diet contributes to cancer. The study also shows a low-carb, paleo diet is an effective treatment for cancer."[6] Whole grains have been touted as an antioxidant, and they may be; however, all grains can elevate your insulin levels, including whole grains. It's all about the glucose. Elevated insulin levels can increase your risk of chronic disease. Excess glucose feeds tumor cells, and insulin drives the propagation of cancerous tissue. Grains can be quite bad because they tend to increase inflammation and deplete nutrient provisions. Inflammation worsens many diseases, cancer included.

What about gluten? There is increasing awareness about the effects of gluten in the diet. Gluten is the protein found in the grain of wheat, barley, and rye. It is essentially the sticky substance that holds bread dough together and establishes its texture. The growing awareness of gluten sensitivity and allergies can have a profound impact on health. Many people have an issue with gluten and do not know it. I read recently on a box of gluten-free product that they now estimate as much as 50 percent of the population may be gluten intolerant. I've read recently that some believe the prominent use of the herbicide glyphosate is causing gut damage leading to gluten sensitivities and allergies (GMO food). If true, virtually everyone will eventually have issues with gluten. Those with gluten issues tend to have difficulty absorbing nutrients, quite possibly leading to illness and/or disease progression.

After requesting the blood test in 2009, I was found to be allergic to gluten. Once I cut it out of my diet, my stomach pains and severe acid reflux disappeared. Symptoms can vary and may include an itchy skin rash, diarrhea, constipation, and digestive issues like stomach pains, especially after a meal. Symptoms that you may experience but are unlikely to be considered include brain fog, autoimmune dysfunction, chronic fatigue, neurological symptoms, hormone imbalance, infertility, fibromyalgia, anxiety, and depression. With celiac disease (an allergy to gluten), the small fibers of the small intestine that absorb nutrients are damaged and certain digestive enzymes are no longer available to aid in digestion. The intestinal wall can become permeable (leaky gut syndrome), and this damage can lead to serious health implications. If you have an allergy or intolerance to gluten, you have the option to switch to ready-made gluten-free products for making breads, pizza, and desserts.

Please keep in mind, however, that these products are carbohydrates and likely to be highly refined. Assuming that they are good for you may be a leap. Simply avoiding products that normally contain gluten may be best for your overall health. Continuing to eat gluten when you have an allergy or intolerance can lead to nutritional deficiency, compromised immune function, and/or intestinal cancer.

The link between high-carb diets and the risk for breast cancer is an emerging area of research. "A particular study enrolled 475 women newly diagnosed with breast cancer and a comparison group of 1,391 healthy women in Mexico City who were matched for age, weight, childbirth trends and other factors that affect the odds of getting the disease. Those in the top category who consumed 62 percent or more of their calories from carbs, were 2.22 times more likely to have breast cancer than those in the lowest category, whose carb intake was 52 percent or less of their diet."[7]

A 2011 study suggests that high dietary glycemic index is associated with a significantly increased risk of breast cancer.[8] How a food affects your insulin levels can be found in the food's glycemic index. The goal of the GI is to measure the change in blood glucose levels after consuming a particular food; the higher the index, the more negative the effect on blood glucose. The glycemic index rating categorizes food based on a scale of zero to 100, with 100 referring to pure glucose. If you take into consideration the quantity of carbohydrate being consumed, you can calculate the glycemic load or total impact. Watermelon interestingly will have a higher glycemic index but lower glycemic load per serving. A lower glycemic index can be found in fructose or fruit sugar than table sugar but, by contrast, will carry a higher glycemic load per serving. Pay close attention to not only what you are eating, but how much and in what combination. Additionally, it may be useful to note that the riper the fruit, the higher the fructose level, so a GI chart may not be accurate for all occasions.

Both of these glycemic measurements are determined by the carbohydrate content of the food. A serving of meat, for instance, will have nil carbohydrate content while providing a high protein intake. Interestingly, up to 50 percent of that protein may be converted to glucose when there is little or no carbohydrate consumed with it. So you need not feel compelled to eat bread or a roll to fulfill your bodies need for carbohydrates. Diabetics have a pretty good handle on this thought process, as it directly relates to their daily living. The American Diabetes Association supports the glycemic index but warns that the "total amount of carbohydrate in the food is still the strongest and most important factor, and that everyone should determine their own custom eating plan that works best for them."[9]

So by paying attention to how you feel after eating certain carbohydrate-rich foods, you can become more aware of the impact of them on your body. After eating pancakes for breakfast with sugary syrup, for example, you may notice hunger coming on faster and more urgently, a few hours later. You may even get light-headed when your blood sugar levels start to crash. Having a high glycemic index and load, this type of food will digest quickly, releasing glucose rapidly into the bloodstream. Foods will tend to have a low glycemic index when they break down more slowly and release glucose in a gradual manner. In general, foods closer to the source, such as nuts, seeds, and plant-based foods, are going to have a low glycemic index

(<55). Higher indexes (>70) will be found in the simple, processed carbohydrates, such as white bread and rice, bagels, and breakfast cereal.

Here's a general guideline to the glycemic index:[10]

Glycemic Indes Overview of what's high and low in Glycemic Index		
Classification	RI Range	Examples
Low GI	55 or Less	Most fruits and Vegetables (except potatoes, watermelon) grainy bread, brown rice, fish, egg
Medium GI	56-69	Whole wheat products, basmati rice, sweet potato, table sugar, white rice.
High GI	70 or more	Flakes, rice krispies, baked potatoes, white bread, straight glucose (100)

© www.medindia.net

There will be a difference, for example, between choosing whole-wheat spaghetti and instant rice. By choosing a carbohydrate source that is rich in nutrients and understanding its impact on bodily systems, you can make a significant impact on your health. There are helpful GI calculators available online that provide a value when you input a food source.

What you can do: Start by adding foods (and equivalents) from the low glycemic index category, perhaps three per week, while reducing or avoiding the foods listed in the high glycemic index category. Transfer carbohydrate choices from the more refined to whole grain, and then reduce the portion size of them. You will be the best judge on quantity reduction based on your current consumption. Continued improvement should be your goal. Keep in mind that all foods are not listed, but the more processed the food, generally, the more quickly it will break down and the higher the GI.

The Food Pyramid

The Great Depression of the 1930s produced a variety of legislation giving the USDA (US Department of Agriculture) new authority. The purpose of this new authority was to boost falling agricultural prices while helping to feed the poor. The USDA needed to solve the problem of abundant product as well as the low price of that product. They contended authority to set nutrition policy when it publicly declared that the purpose of the surplus food program was to "dispose of surplus food and simultaneously raise the nutritional level of low-income consumers."[11]

Every five to seven years since 1933, the US Congress passes legislation acts known as the Farm Bill. The Farm Bill includes subsidies to growers of certain types of food. The top four most subsidized foods are corn, soybeans, wheat, and rice. The original Food Pyramid, which I was taught in school, had grains as the largest bottom block of the pyramid, encouraging you to eat six to eleven servings of bread, cereal, rice, and pasta a day.

It would seem that from the beginning, USDA dietary guidelines may have been based more on what farmers have and need to sell than what your body requires to stay healthy. The pyramid was replaced in 2005, followed by My Plate in 2011. Although an improvement, the new guideline has removed virtually all fats from the equation, despite advances in nutritional science confirming that nonprocessed, healthy fats are an important staple to good health.

Dairy

"Milk, no surprise, is pretty nutritious. It's got protein, a bunch of micronutrients, lots of calcium and plenty of carbohydrates. 'For the ancient Neolithic Farmer, it was a superfood,' says Mark Thomas, an evolutionary geneticist at University College London in the U.K."[12] Today, there is much skepticism regarding the overall value of consuming dairy products. Thought to be very different than the milk of our ancestors, it is seen by many to be highly inflammatory—a symptom to be avoided for many reasons, including cancer prevention.

Dr. Ben Kim, a holistic practitioner, states three important facts you should know about most varieties of milk that are widely available in grocery stores. "First of all, cows are fed high-protein soybean meal and growth hormones to increase production. Both increase a cow's risk of health issues leading to frequent doses of antibiotics. Secondly, conventional milk is pasteurized, exposing it to high temperatures resulting in denaturing proteins, making them less usable and even harmful to your body. Pasteurization also destroys enzymes, one of which helps your body absorb the calcium. It destroys vitamins B12, B6, and C while also destroying friendly bacteria. Thirdly, many varieties of milk are homogenized which can alter healthy fat and cholesterol in a way that leaves them more susceptible to forming free radicals, a potential cancer precursor."[13]

Realmilk.com is a website that provides nutrition education on what constitutes healthy milk and where to find it. Even if you do find it, it may be possible that it is still not a healthy choice for you. "Many people have difficulty digesting casein, a major protein found in milk. Ongoing exposure to casein that is not properly broken down is strongly associated with chronic ear infections, nasal congestion, acne, eczema, a variety of autoimmune illnesses, and even cancer."[13]

If you happen to be of the O blood type, which is the predominant blood type, you may have an allergy or intolerance to dairy. Type O is the oldest blood type, according to Dr. Peter J. D'Adamo and Catherine Whitney, authors of *Eat Right for Your Type.* "Their system is ill designed for … proper metabolism [of dairy products]," Dr. D'Adamo explains, "and those with blood type O should severely restrict their use of dairy products. Early man was a hunter-gatherer, thriving on meat, killing any big game to be found within their hunting range. If you are of type 'O' and do eat incorrectly, your risk factors for ulcers and inflammatory diseases such as arthritis increase." If you are this type and prone to arthritis, you may wish to obtain the full list of advisable avoidances. "If you are of the blood type 'A,' or 'AB,' he advises that you also avoid dairy products. If you are type 'A' and eat incorrectly, your risk factors for cancer and heart disease are said to increase. Blood type 'B' is the only blood type that does well with dairy."[14]

A study done by Kaiser Permanente researchers and published online by the *Journal of the National Cancer Institute* on March 14, 2013, suggests that women diagnosed with early-stage breast cancer who eat full-fat dairy products after diagnosis are more likely to die from breast cancer than women who eat low-fat dairy products after diagnosis.[15] The reason may be the very thing that makes a woman feel feminine—estrogen. "The hormone estrogen stimulates breast cell growth, including the growth of hormone-receptor-positive breast cancer cells." Estrogen is not just produced by the ovaries. "It is also created and stored in fat cells. Many researchers believe that dairy products eaten in the United States and other Western countries have high levels of estrogen and progesterone in them because most of the milk is produced by pregnant cows. So it might be possible that low-fat dairy products have lower levels of estrogen and progesterone because most of the fat has been removed. This suggests that low-fat dairy products may be a better choice for women who've been diagnosed with breast cancer, especially hormone-receptor-positive breast cancer."[16]

Jane Plant, author of *Your Life in Your Hands*, claims that eliminating dairy products from her diet saved her from dying of breast cancer, which recurred five times. She argues that a person can prevent such a diagnosis or recurrence by doing the same. "Cow's milk is a perfect food for a rapidly growing baby calf," she writes, but "cow's milk isn't intended by nature for consumption by any species other than baby cows."[17]

What you can do: If you are not already doing so, avoid dairy when possible, keeping in mind that the more you consume, the greater the possibility of increased inflammation and discomfort. Low-temperature pasteurization is available in some areas. If you simply love dairy and are not willing to abstain, consider consuming a low-fat variety and/or researching and obtaining healthy milk to mitigate the potential negative effects. Also, for eating dairy occasionally, a digestive enzyme taken with first bite may be helpful. Discuss calcium supplementation with your doctor.

Meat

While working on my undergraduate degree, I attended a private Seventh-day Adventist university due to convenience and its close proximity. Those of the Seventh-day Adventist faith tend to follow a well-balanced vegetarian diet with some eating a lacto-ovo vegetarian diet, which allows for milk and eggs but no animal flesh. There was a dairy farm on campus, but I do not know their views on pasteurization or homogenization. The Adventists have followed this diet to honor and glorify God for more than a century. Interestingly, a multitude of studies have proven "most of these individuals to be healthier than the general population. Seventh-day Adventists have a 50% lower risk of developing heart disease, certain types of cancers, strokes, and diabetes. "A study of Seventh-day Adventists published in 2000 showed that the 34,192 self-identified California Adventists who were followed for 12 years lived, on average, 7.3 extra years for men and 4.42 more years for women, when compared to other non-Hispanic Californians.

The Seventh-day Adventist diet also recommends abstinence from alcohol, coffee, tea, and all other caffeinated beverages. Lacto-ovo vegetarians need to pay special attention to what they eat to make sure that they get enough iron, zinc, and protein from their diet. Total vegetarians should pay close attention to calcium, vitamin B12, iron, zinc, and protein. It is recommended that people choose plain and simply prepared foods whenever possible. The Adventist eating plan focuses on choosing whole-grain and high-fiber foods, while minimizing the simple, high glycemic index carbohydrates."[18]

According to the Physicians Committee on Responsible Medicine, "there is a growing consensus showing a connection between meat consumption and cancer risk. First, they claim, meat devoid of fiber and the nutrients which provide a protective effect again cancer. Meat also contains animal protein, saturated fat, and, in some cases, carcinogenic compounds such as heterocyclic amines (HCA) and polycyclic aromatic hydrocarbons (PAH) formed during the processing or cooking of meat."[19]

In 2007 a major cancer research institute published its second review of the major studies on food, nutrition, and cancer prevention. "For cancers of the esophagus, lung, pancreas, stomach, colon or rectum, endometrium, and prostate, it was determined that red meat (beef, pork, or lamb) and processed meat consumption possibly increased cancer risk. For colorectal cancer, a review of the literature determined that there is convincing scientific evidence that red meat increased cancer risk and that processed meat, saturated/animal fat, and heavily cooked meat were also convincing of increased risk."[20]

Then in 2015, after thoroughly reviewing the accumulated scientific literature, a Working Group of twenty-two experts from ten countries convened by the International Agency for Research on Cancer (IARC), the cancer agency of the World Health Organization, Monographs Program classified "the consumption of red meat as probably carcinogenic to humans, based on limited evidence that the consumption of red meat causes cancer in humans and strong mechanistic evidence supporting a carcinogenic effect."[21]

A study in the *British Journal of Cancer* found that "vegetarians are 12 percent less likely to develop cancer than meat-eaters. After following 61,000 meat eaters and vegetarians for over 12 years, researchers also discovered that cancers of the blood—such as leukemia, multiple myeloma, and non-Hodgkin lymphoma—were drastically reduced by as much as 45 percent for those following a vegetarian diet. Although this study points to an overall reduced risk, this may well be an underestimate of the benefit of a vegetarian diet. Although pancreatic cancer may seem to be the cancer most negatively affected by meat and dairy consumption, studies have shown up to a 40% decrease in all cancers by following a vegetarian diet."[22]

To avoid Heterocyclic Amines (HCAs), the chemicals formed when muscle meat is cooked via high-temperature methods, do the following:

- Cook at lower temperatures
- Keep your grill clean by scraping off charred residue

- Trim fat and remove skin before cooking
- Don't cook directly over heat source, coals, or flame; increase distance from heat source
- Use leaner cuts to reduce flaming
- Use a marinade

What you can do: Avoid processed meat like bacon and smoked sausage. If you are a meat eater and find it a difficult food choice to give up, consider using organic lean cuts of meat and avoid high heat and overcooking. If you enjoy grilling, be aware that you are potentially producing cancer-causing chemicals called heterocyclic amines (HCA). The blackened or charred areas of the meat are the source, initiating a mutation that can lead to cancer. You might also consider reducing your portion size. Eliminating the need to have meat as the main staple for your meal might be an option to consider. Eating more casseroles, like scalloped potatoes with ham, with smaller amounts of meat can help you during the transition.

Soy

There is an array of information currently flying around regarding the benefits and harmfulness of soy. If you are confused, join the crowd. *Vibrant Life* magazine calls the soybean the miracle bean.[23] Soybeans seem to contain high levels of several compounds with demonstrated anticancer activity. For example, soybeans are very rich in unique sources of isoflavonoids, such as genistein. There are claims that these isoflavonoids have been shown to inhibit the growth of human breast cancer cells. There are doctors, however, including Dr. Mercola, who claim otherwise. "The phytoestrogen genistein, naturally found in soybeans, has been found to heighten the estrogenic effects of glyphosate, prompting the warning that genetically engineered soybeans may therefore pose a breast cancer risk. According to Dr. Mercola, these compounds mimic and sometimes block the hormone estrogen, and have been found to have adverse effects on various human tissues. Soy phytoestrogens are known to disrupt endocrine function, may cause infertility, and may promote breast cancer in women."[24] It would seem that the very characteristics that are deemed healthful by some are deemed detrimental by others. This is why doing your own research and determining what information resonates with you is so important.

The real confusion regarding soy seems to culminate with one criterion: Is it fermented or not? Soy is, indeed, big business— very big business. "From 2000 to 2007, U.S. food manufacturers introduced more than 2,700 new soy-based foods, and new soy products continue to appear on your grocer's shelves. And as of 2007, 85 percent of consumers perceived soy products as healthful."[24]

Dr. Kaayla Daniel, author of *The Whole Soy Story*, points out "thousands of studies linking soy to malnutrition, digestive distress, immune-system breakdown, thyroid dysfunction, cognitive decline, reproductive disorders and infertility—even cancer and heart disease. These are just a sample of the health effects that have been linked to soy consumption."[25]

Soy can be incredibly healthful but should be considered only when it is organic and properly fermented. After fermentation, the phytate and antinutrient levels of soybeans are reduced, and their beneficial properties become available to your digestive system. This is the fundamental difference in the value of soy consumption. All soy is not created equal.

Soy products to avoid:

- Tofu
- TVP (texturized vegetable protein)
- Soybean oil

- Soy milk
- Soy cheese
- Soy protein
- Edamame
- Soy infant formula

Fermented soy products to consider:

- Tempeh, a fermented soybean cake with a firm texture and nutty, mushroom-like flavor
- Miso, a fermented soybean paste with a salty, buttery texture (commonly used in miso soup)
- Natto, fermented soybeans with a sticky texture and strong, cheese-like flavor
- Soy sauce, which is traditionally made by fermenting soybeans, salt and enzymes; be wary because many varieties on the market today are made artificially using a chemical process

For years we have been told that soy is healthful and beneficial. It appears that we have been misled yet again. In time and with more research, we can hope to be more fully and uniformly informed. It makes you wonder which establishment can benefit from totally misguided information.

What you can do: Read labels carefully and make good choices. Products made with soy ingredients have taken the food industry by storm. It can be found in packaged foods like bouillon, baking mixes, energy bars, peanut butter, mayonnaise, and chocolate, to name a few.

The Macrobiotic Approach

There seems to be some truth to that old adage, "You are what you eat." Have you been hearing more and more about the importance of nutrition for the treatment and prevention of cancer? For example, The Cancer Treatment Centers of America are using a more holistic approach by providing critical nutritional therapy to their patients along with traditional treatment methodologies. I have personally heard some amazing stories about those who have chosen nutrition over what would be considered today to be standard cancer treatment: surgery, chemotherapy, and radiation. I look forward to the day when these latter medical traditions will be considered inhuman and archaic.

One such amazing story involved the macrobiotic diet. In the early nineties, the mother of a friend was diagnosed with breast cancer. The diagnosis itself can be traumatic leaving one in shock and disbelief. It would be reasonable and customary to follow the direction of the doctors and specialists with standard, mainstream treatment. Injecting the body with harsh chemicals, dangerous to major systems and organs of the body, seems problematic. These chemicals also generate the potential to cause another cancer: leukemia. They may be considered financially healthy in that they maintain a prominent need and lifestyle for many an oncologist.

But my friend's mother cleared her head and looked at other options. When faced with life-altering decisions, an open mind is essential to good judgment. I am certainly not saying that traditional medicine is not the best choice for you. Steve Jobs chose alternative treatment, and in his final days, he regretted it. Education is the key. I am simply encouraging you to review all options and make a decision that you feel is best for you. You may feel like a statistic, but I assure you that you are not. You are a beautifully and wonderfully made individual, different than every other soul in the universe. What you choose may not be the same as what someone else would choose, and that is okay. In the end, after careful consideration, the choice you make for you is the best choice.

According to Wikipedia, the macrobiotic diet is a dietary regimen that involves eating complex grains as a staple food, supplemented with other foods, such as local vegetables, while avoiding the use of highly processed or refined foods and most animal products. Webster's is less descriptive, stating that it's a diet consisting mainly of beans and whole grains.

Perhaps you have heard that it is best to shop the outside walls of the grocery store and avoid the center aisles. In doing so, you are buying more basic nutrition, closer to the source, like produce, and not buying the processed products or boxed foods. The macrobiotic diet also addresses the manner of eating by recommending against overeating and by encouraging that food be chewed thoroughly.

"Followers of the traditional macrobiotic approach believe that food and food quality powerfully affect health, well-being, and happiness, and that a traditional locally based macrobiotic diet has more beneficial effects than others."[26] Again, the modern macrobiotic approach suggests choosing food that is less processed. Choosing food as medicine may be the best decision one can make.

Cancer rates vary dramatically between countries, none more so than between Japan and the United States. Overall age-adjusted cancer rates in the United States are more than 50 percent higher than in Japan. If you were to create a food pyramid that depicts the guidelines for the Japanese-style macrobiotic diet, the bottom-most compartment would be well-chewed whole cereal grains, especially brown rice, at 40 percent of daily calories. The next compartment above grains would be vegetables at 25 to 30 percent. Above vegetables would be 5 to 10 percent beans and legumes. Next would be miso soup, sea vegetables, and traditionally or naturally processed foods at 5 percent each. To top off the pyramid, you would have the small amounts of fish, seafood, seeds, nuts, seasonings, sweeteners, fruits, and beverages to be enjoyed two to three times per week.

A German study conducted in 2012 evaluated several diets, including the Budwig Diet, Gerson's regiment, the low-carb diet, the Breuss Cancer Cure, and the microbiotic diet. The Gerson diet is an approach that utilizes organic foods, supplementation, and detox protocols to heal the body as a whole. A rigid diet is the core of the Breuss Cancer Cure, consisting of fasting combined with special vegetable juices and teas. The study methodology analyzed chat rooms for cancer patients using the search engines Google and Bing. Then using their own counseling experience as experts, they conducted systematic literature review of clinical data in Medline. They indicated that they did not find any scientific publication of a clinical study that describes positive results toward survival.

Based on my research, it is my opinion that these diets may be quite helpful for healing a cancerous condition or for keeping cancer at arm's length. I will leave it to you to determine if this is the best method to conduct research and reach a morally respectable conclusion. I would encourage you to dig deeper when you hear a medical news headline and analyze the testing population, how the study was performed, how many participated, and, most importantly, who funded the study. If you are in a place where you want to change your nutritional habits and eat more whole foods, do your *own* research and decide what nutritional genre feels best to you. You may need to do an aggressive program for a short time to jump-start your healing, but ultimately, you want to make changes that are sustainable.

I found it interesting that the American Cancer Society does not endorse the macrobiotic diet, claiming it to be without scientific proof. The American Cancer Society's nutritional guidelines recommend eating a balanced diet that includes five or more servings a day of vegetables and fruit, choosing whole grains over processed and refined foods, and limiting red meats and animal fats. They feel that it is best to choose foods from a variety of fruits, vegetables, and other plant sources such as nuts, seeds, whole-grain cereals, and beans to take in all needed nutrients. In my unprofessional opinion, their recommendations seem much in line with the macrobiotic diet with the exception of allowing small amounts of meat. But by all indications, my friend's mother reduced her cancer tumor and remains healthy by maintaining the utilization of the macrobiotic diet.

Food's Estrogen Load

Dr. Bob Arnot discusses *The Breast Cancer Prevention Diet* in his book of the same name. He notes that "breast cancer could take as long as 33 years to develop and for much of that time it is unseen and undetectable, in fact, only when a tumor reaches one billion cells in size can a mammogram detect it. That's the smallest size that a radiologist can see but is simply enormous in terms of cancer growth. The best prevention is to interfere with cancer's ability to generate and replicate."[27]

According to a 2001 Applied Nutritional Science report, "many nutrients effectively reduce estrogen load by supporting preferred pathways of estrogen metabolism and detoxification. These include indole-3 carbinol, B vitamins, magnesium, calcium D-glucarate, flax seed, phytonutrients like curcumin, and antioxidants. The influence of these nutrients on estrogen metabolism may have profound significance for diseases and conditions in which estrogen plays a role in clinical expression."[28]

In a 2002 report published in *Alternative Medicine Review*, investigators analyzed the available research on calcium D-glucarate and found that it may inhibit beta-glucuronidase (an enzyme associated with increased risk for various hormone-dependent cancers when it occurs at elevated levels). "Calcium D-glucarate is the calcium salt of D-glucaric acid, produced naturally in small amounts by mammals, including humans. Glucaric acid is found in fruits and vegetables with the highest concentrations to be found in oranges, apples, grapefruit, and cruciferous vegetables."[29]

Speaking for myself, when my estrogen metabolism was found to be at unhealthy levels, I started a supplement regiment of DIM-CDG. (diiindolymethane with calcium D-glucarate). Research may be limited, but my results were very positive. Diindolylmethane is a natural substance produced when the body breaks down indole-3-carbinol (a compound found in cruciferous vegetables, such as broccoli and cauliflower). "Diindolylmethane is purported to produce changes in estrogen metabolism, a biological process thought to influence the development of certain hormone-dependent cancers, such as breast cancer."[30]

"Taking a DIM supplement is like consuming large quantities of cruciferous vegetables. Studies, while sometimes inconclusive, support the intake of cruciferous vegetables for the prevention of breast cancer."[31] US researchers at the Roswell Park Cancer Institute found the following:

> The intake of cruciferous vegetables in premenopausal women was inversely associated with the risk of breast cancer. The researchers concluded that cruciferous vegetables may play an important role in decreasing the risk of premenopausal breast cancer.

> Cruciferous vegetables contain sulfur-rich glucosinolates that need to go through an enzymatic reaction before producing the cancer fighting I3C and DIM. The enzyme that does this is called myrosinase, which is actually part of cruciferous vegetables. When you cut or chew a cruciferous vegetable the enzyme comes in contact with

the glucosinolates, starting the formation process of I3C and DIM. DIM is actually two I3C molecules connected together during the digestive process.

Unfortunately, various factors may reduce the cancer fighting potency of cruciferous vegetables. Boiling, steaming, and microwaving can reduce the activity of the myrosinase enzyme. Because glucosinolates are water soluble they are readily leeched into the water when cruciferous vegetables are boiled, reducing their content up to 58 percent. Due to these factors, eating cruciferous vegetables raw or lightly sautéing them will maximize the amount of I3C and DIM that may be formed.

Providentially, dietary supplements of I3C and DIM can provide high levels of these potent nutrients in a single and convenient capsule, wherein one capsule contains far more I3C and DIM than a serving of cruciferous vegetables."[2]

You will find additional information in chapter four of this book, which focuses on supplementation.

Additional Sustenance of High-Consequence

Vitamin C

There are several clinics in the United States that use high-dose intravenous vitamin C (IVC) treatment to treat cancer cells.[33] If high doses can be used to treat cancer, could smaller doses be effective for prevention? By 1991 approximately ninety epidemiologic studies had examined the role of vitamin C or vitamin-C-rich foods in cancer prevention, and the vast majority found statistically significant protective effects. Regarding breast cancer specifically, evidence points to a consistent and significant protective effect of elevated dietary vitamin C intake.[34, 35]

Vitamin C is a water-soluble vitamin, meaning that your body does not store it. The body will use what it needs and then excrete the leftover amounts via the urine. It has other names, such as ascorbic acid or dehydroascorbic acid (DHAA). "Vitamin C is considered one of many antioxidant nutrients. These are key nutrients that hinder much of the damage caused by free radicals. Free radicals are made when your body breaks down food or when we are exposed to negative environmental elements like cigarette smoke, for example. Free radicals play a role in cancer, heart disease and other conditions."[36]

Fighting free radicals is essential for living in the world we currently find ourselves in; however, vitamin C provides a powerhouse of benefits. "It is required for the synthesis of collagen, a protein that plays a critical role in the structure of our bodies. Collagen is the framework for our skin and our bones, and without it, we would quite literally fall apart. Vitamin C is necessary to make certain neurotransmitters like serotonin, a hormone that plays a critical role in a wide variety of body systems, including nervous system, endocrine system, immune system, and digestive system. Antioxidants in foods tend to work together in important synergistic ways to provide protection against free radical damage."[37] "Vitamin C also has intrinsic antiviral and antibacterial activity and is beneficial in general immunity boosting, helping to ward off or prevent colds and flus, assisting the healing of wounds, aiding the body in fighting infection."[38]

Because our bodies cannot produce vitamin C on their own and cannot store it, it is essential that we maintain a consistent habit of eating foods containing plenty of vitamin C. Colorful foods may be an indication of a nutrient-rich food source. You may be surprised to learn that a half cup of sweet red pepper contains more vitamin C than an orange. This would be in its raw form, keeping in mind that water-soluble nutrients may have reduced nutritional content when cooked (heated).

Here is an example of optimal food sources for vitamin C:[39]

Food	Serving	mg	% DV
red pepper, sweet, raw	1/2 cup	95	158
orange juice	3/4 cup	93	155
orange	1 medium	70	117
grapefruit juice	3/4 cup	70	117
kiwifruit	1 medium	64	107
green pepper, sweet, raw	1/2 cup	60	100
broccoli, cooked	1/2 cup	51	85
strawberries, sliced	1/2 cup	49	82
Brussels sprouts, cooked	1/2 cup	48	80
grapefruit	1/2 medium	39	65
broccoli, raw	1/2 cup	39	65
tomato juice	3/4 cup	33	55
cantaloupe	1/2 cup	29	48
cabbage, cooked	1/2 cup	28	47
cauliflower, raw	1/2 cup	26	43
potato, baked	1 medium	17	28
tomato, raw	1 medium	17	28
spinach	1/2 cup	9	15
green peas, frozen, cooked	1/2 cup	8	13

And even when you can partake of nutrient-rich vitamin C food sources, supplementation could be considered. Ascorbic acid is the synthetic version of vitamin C and not considered a living complex. It is a copy of a part of a living complex known as vitamin C. Ascorbic acid is a fractionated, crystalline isolate of vitamin C.[40] Fruits and vegetables are rich in numerous micronutrients, dietary fiber, and phytochemicals like bioflavonoids and should be considered your primary source of vitamin C—food derived. The presence of these bonus features may affect the nutritional absorption of vitamin C. Eating plenty of foods dense with vitamin C should be your priority.

Two-time Nobel Prize winner, Dr. Linus Pauling was the first to realize vitamin C's crucial importance in the maintenance of a healthy immune system. In 1970 he proposed that regular intake of vitamin C in amounts far higher than the officially sanctioned recommended daily allowance, and many experts are now realizing that the RDA is far too low to provide optimum health and protection against disease. "A team of medical researchers at the National Institutes of Health in the USA completed a study designed to determine the vitamin C requirements of healthy, young men. They found that a minimum intake of 1000 mg/day was required to completely saturate the blood plasma with vitamin C. They also found that vitamin C should be taken in divided doses throughout the day as urinary excretion increases rapidly when individual doses exceed 500 mg."[41,42]

An independent testing company has determined that "vitamin C is not accurately listed on 27% of supplements," so if you decide to buy a supplement, do your research.[43] Because it can be acidic, a buffered version, with magnesium, calcium, potassium, etc., may be a better choice. Buffered vitamin C, derived from beets, is known to be gentler on the stomach than ascorbic acid, which is derived from corn. Either way, you may want to be sure that it is GMO free.

Your best bet, as we have discussed, may be to consume five or more servings of fruits and vegetables per day; however, many Americans are not willing and/or able to consume such a diet.

Zinc

We can take supplemental zinc as discussed in chapter 4, but as we've discussed, food is the optimum option for nutrients. Zinc is an essential mineral that is naturally present in some foods, added to others, and available as a dietary supplement. As we have discussed, "deficiency of zinc is prevalent worldwide most especially in developing countries and may affect nearly 2 billion subjects."[44] "In the US currently 50% of men and women age 50 and older are consuming less than the RDA, 11 and 9 mg respectively, with 10% consuming less than one half of the recommended amount."[45] "Like vitamin C, the body has no specialized zinc storage system, therefore, daily intake is required to maintain numerous aspects of cellular metabolism. It plays a role in immune function, protein synthesis, DNA synthesis, cell division, and catalytic activity of approximately 100 enzymes."[46, 47]

Because animal products seem to contain the highest amounts, the majority of Americans get most of their zinc from meat and poultry. Phytates in whole grains will bind with zinc and inhibit its absorption. Because vegetarians omit meat from their diets and commonly eat a lot of legumes and whole grains, they may require up to 50 percent more than the recommended daily allowance for zinc than those who eat meat.

The food sources with the highest amounts of zinc include shellfish and muscle meats, with oysters being at the top of the list. Select food sources for zinc include:[48]

Food	Serving	mg	%DV
oysters, cooked	3 oz	74	493
beef, chuck roast	3 oz	7	47
crab, Alaskan king, cooked	3 oz	6.5	43
beef patty, broiled	3 oz	5.3	35
cereal, fortified	3/4 cup	3.8	25
lobster	3 oz	3.4	23
pork chop, loin, cooked	3 oz	2.9	19
baked beans, canned	1/2 cup	2.9	19
chicken, dark meat, cooked	3 oz	2.4	16
yogurt, fruit, low fat	8 oz	1.7	11
cashews, dry roasted	1 oz	1.6	11
chickpeas, cooked	1/2 cup	1.3	9
cheese, Swiss	1 oz	1.2	8
oatmeal, instant, plain	1 packet	1.1	7
milk, low-fat	1 cup	1	7
almonds, dry roasted	1 oz	0.9	6
kidney beans, cooked	1/2 cup	0.9	6
peas, green, frozen, cooked	1/2 cup	0.5	3
founder or sole, cooked	3 oz	0.3	2

Other food sources include "brewer's yeast, egg yolks, kelp, lamb, lima beans, liver, mushrooms, pecans, pumpkin seeds, sardines, and sunflower seeds. Zinc is also found in alfalfa, curdock, cayenne, chamomile, dandelion, eyebright, fennel seeds, milk thistle, nettle, parsley, rose hips, sage, skullcap, and wild yam."[49]

"Many studies are now addressing the importance of the proper intake of dietary nutrients in the prevention of cancer. Among them, zinc has been found to play a pivotal role in host defense against the initiation and promotion of several malignancies."[50] "In a 2009 study conducted at Wayne State University School of Medicine, Detroit, the patient's zinc status was a better indicator of tumor burden and stage of disease in comparison to the overall nutritional status. The researcher concluded that zinc supplementation should have beneficial effects on cancer by decreasing the formation and differentiation of blood vessels, decreasing the induction of inflammatory proteins while increasing apoptosis (the genetically directed process of cell self-destruction) in cancer cells."[51]

Zinc may be a key mineral in the fight against breast cancer. "The primary gene protecting women from breast cancer, p53, is thought to be the most frequently mutated or altered gene in the development of cancer. This gene requires zinc, and if it is missing, the gene becomes mutated, resulting in it becoming inactivated or suppressed. Dysfunction of p53 is well documented in the development of breast cancer, indicating that a zinc deficiency is a risk factor for breast cancer."[52]

So it would seem that we are not consuming the proper foods and/ or amounts of the right foods to maintain healthy levels of zinc in our bodies. Supplementation should be considered. "Zinc is not easily absorbed in the body unless 'chelated' or first attached to another substance. Zinc Orotate is zinc that has been chelated to orotic acid. This form contains many antioxidant properties that can help protect your health, while offering your cells a readily-absorbable form of zinc. Zinc Picolinate is a form that has been chelated to picolinic amino acids. One of the most popular forms, zinc gluconate, is just a chemical form of zinc that is created by a process of industrial manufacturing. Zinc Acetate for zinc salt dehydrate is created by adding acetic acid to zinc carbonate or zinc metal. Zinc Sulfate is a water-soluble and non-chelated, inorganic form of zinc."[53]

"Because there is no specific bodily system for zinc storage, it is regulated tightly with 98% of the body's supply within the cells at any given time. This system makes zinc levels very difficult to measure using laboratory methods. There is, however, a DIY taste test kit, first reported by the medical journal, The Lancet. This particular do-it-yourself kit can help determine physiological zinc levels. This test uses Premier Research Labs, Liquid Zinc Assay, an easily absorbed form of supplemental zinc sulfate heptahydrate. If you are deficient in zinc, the liquid will taste like water, while if you have adequate levels, it will taste bitter."[54]

Selenium

Another important mineral in the breast cancer prevention tool kit is selenium. "It is considered nutritional essential to humans with critical roles in reproduction, thyroid hormone metabolism, DNA synthesis, while protecting from oxidative damage and infection."[55] The selenium content in our foods can be closely linked with the content found in the soils. Brazil nuts are considered a good source of selenium. One ounce of this nut may contain as much as ten times the recommended daily amount. The current RDA for selenium is 55 mcg. Certain food groups are generally considered higher in sources of selenium. Here are some examples:[56]

Food	Serving	mcg	%DV
tuna	4 oz	122	223
Brazil nut	1 nut	95	172
shrimp	4 oz	56	102
salmon	4 oz	43	78
cod	4 oz	31	58
cremini mushrooms	1 cup	18	34

shiitake mushrooms	1/2 cup	18	33
asparagus	1 cup	11	20
mustard seeds	2 tsp	8	15
turkey	4 oz	34	62
chicken	4 oz	31	57
lamb	4 oz	27	51
scallops	4 oz	24	45
beef	4 oz	24	44
barley	1/3 cup	23	42
eggs	1 egg	15	36
brown rice	1 cup	19	35
sunflower seeds	1/4 cup	18	34
sesame seeds	1/4 cup	12	23

If you tend to follow a vegetarian or vegan diet, you may be low in selenium. Of other consideration is any condition associated with malabsorption, like celiac disease, for example. It is also important to note that "serum selenium concentrations tend to decline with age. This downward inclination in selenium concentrations might be associated with age-related declines in brain function, possibly due to selenium's antioxidant activity."[57]

In the United States we tend to lack selenium in our diet simply because it is typically processed out of standard fare. The following ailments are some conditions that may signal a deficit in selenium: high cholesterol, persistent infections, weakened liver, exhaustion, and lack of pancreatic enzymes for digestion.

"In 2009, a study was done in the Klang Valley, an area in Malaysia which is centered in Kuala Lumpur. The purpose of the study was to assess the relationship between selenium status and intake among breast cancer patients. Participants ranged in age and ethnicity with their selenium status determined from toenail and hair analysis. Their conclusion: Selenium intake and status was associated with breast cancer risk."[58]

There are various methods you may use to determine current selenium levels. "The most common used measures of selenium status are plasma and serum selenium concentrations."[59] These concentrations in blood and urine will reflect most recent selenium intake. One can analyze hair and or nail samples to monitor longer-term intake over months or years.

As with other key nutrients, it is best to obtain your optimum levels through proper food choices. "Long term consumption of high doses of selenium can lead to complications such as gastrointestinal upsets, hair loss, white blotchy nails, garlic breath odor, fatigue, irritability, and mild nerve damage."[60] If you are concerned that even with proper food choices, you are not achieving a necessary selenium serum level, ask your doctor to perform testing for verification before beginning a supplemental regimen.

Flaxseed

Flax is grown as a food crop in cooler regions of the world. This particular therapeutic plant is native to the area extending from the eastern Mediterranean through Western Asia and the Middle East to India with Canada currently leading in worldwide production.

"Animal research supports flaxseed's role in suppressing breast cancer. In immunosuppressed mice (thymus removed), flaxseed was capable of suppressing the estrogen-fed growth of transplanted human breast cancer tumors. Flaxseed does not just suppress estradiol production, as do blockbuster hormone-suppressive chemotherapy drugs like Arimidex, but nudges estradiol metabolism into a positive direction by generating a higher ratio of the beneficial metabolite 2-hydroxyestrone versus the considered more harmful 16-hydroxylestrone."[61]

The Dzudzuana Cave of the Republic of Georgia seems to indicate the use of flax dating back to the Upper Paleolithic period, some thirty thousand years ago. As early as 3000 BC, flaxseed was cultivated in Babylon, ancient Egypt, and China. The straw in the weed, flax fiber, was spun into fabric. In the eighth century, King Charlemagne, a medieval emperor who ruled much of Western Europe, "believed so strongly in the health benefits of flaxseed that he passed laws requiring his subjects to consume it."[62] Now, centuries later, there are experts claiming to have the research to back up what Charles the Great projected.

Although flaxseed contains all sorts of healthy components, it primarily owes its healthy reputation to three of them:

- Omega-3 essential fatty acids, "good" fats that have been shown to have heart-healthy effects. Each tablespoon of ground flaxseed contains about 1.8 grams of plant omega-3s.
- Lignans, which have both plant estrogen and antioxidant qualities. Flaxseed contains 75 to 800 times more lignans than other plant foods.
- Fiber. Flaxseed contains both the soluble and insoluble types.[63]

"Most of the plant lignans in human foods are converted by the intestinal microflora in the upper part of the large bowel to protective compounds. The role of these compounds, particularly in chronic Western diseases gives rise to the idea that food constitutes a viable medicine. Evidence suggests that fiber- and lignan-rich whole-grain cereals, beans, berries, nuts, and various seeds are the main protective foods. Many factors, in addition to diet, such as intestinal microflora, smoking, antibiotics, and obesity affect circulating lignan levels in the body. Lignan-rich diets may be beneficial, particularly if consumed for life. Experimental evidence in animals has shown clear anticarcinogenic effects of flaxseed or pure lignans in many types of cancer. The source of the lignans seems to play a role because other factors in the food obviously participate in the protective effects."[64] Study results are quite promising.

The American Nutrition Association highlighted the importance of this "neglected food," stating that "flaxseed is not only an excellent source of two fatty acids that are essential for human health— linoleic acid and alpha-linolenic acid," but also, "an excellent source of fiber and a good source of minerals and vitamins."[65]

A 2005 study found dietary flaxseed to have the "potential to reduce tumor growth in patients with breast cancer. This study examined, in a randomized double-blind placebo-controlled clinical trial, the effects of dietary flaxseed on tumor biological markers and urinary lignan excretion in postmenopausal patients with newly diagnosed breast cancer."[66]

Consuming flaxseed has also been found to lower cholesterol, prevent hot flashes, improve blood sugar, and protect skin tissue from the damages of radiation. "Women with breast, uterine, and ovarian cancer or endometriosis should ask their doctor before taking flaxseed, because it may act like an estrogen in the body. This nutrient may alter the effects of some prescription and nonprescription medications."[67] Flaxseed is high in fiber, so although unlikely, you should be aware that it may cause flatulence, stomach pains, nausea, constipation, diarrhea, and bloating. Be sure to consume it with plenty of water.

Flaxseed can be acquired quite easily and will typically be found in brown or yellow color. It is usually recommended that you buy the flaxseed whole, because it is more chemically stable. Ground flaxseed has been found to go rancid at room temperature in as little as one week. Because whole seeds can remain whole when digested, consider grinding immediately before consumption. A small coffee grinder is quite handy for this function. There are all sorts of interesting options for consumption. You can sprinkle ground flaxseed on salad, add it to oatmeal and smoothies, and mix it into your meatloaf and/or baking products. I use about 1 tablespoon of ground flaxseed per serving when mixing a smoothie.

Flaxseed can also be used as an egg substitute. Simply grind the flaxseed (or chia) in the coffee grinder, measure out 1 tablespoon, and add it to 3 tablespoons of water. Stir well and then place in refrigerator for fifteen minutes to set.

Wheatgrass

Wheatgrass is a nutrient-rich young grass from the wheat family. It is cultivated from the first true leaf of the stem or seed embryo of the wheat plant. Many sprouted seeds and grains fall into the superfood category, and this is no exception. Wheatgrass contains abundant chlorophyll content, which can help oxygenate your blood. Known as the green pigment in plants, chlorophyll collects light and uses the light to make energy for those plants. "The use of chlorophyll to promote the healing process was first reported nearly 100 years ago."[68] "Chlorophyll binds with toxic metals to hamper absorption, and research has shown it can do the same with some carcinogens."[69] "It protects cells from oxidative damage by eliminating free radicals."[70] Chlorophyll has been shown to have "antiseptic and anti-inflammatory benefits, helps to regulate bowel habits and provides a rapid method of delivery of magnesium, vitamin K, vitamin C, folic acid, iron, calcium and protein."[71]

According to Hippocrates Health Institute, "two ounces of wheatgrass juice has the nutritional equivalent of five pounds of the best raw organic vegetables."[72] When starting a consistent wheatgrass regimen, it is essential to be careful and to start slowly to avoid nausea and stimulation of a healing crisis. You may feel dizzy or lightheaded if you consume too much too quickly. In liquid form, start with one ounce once or twice daily and then transition to two ounces twice a day at your own pace. An alternative option for you is to simply buy liquid chlorophyll at your local health food store and begin adding the suggested amount to water. My resource exhibits minty characteristics, and I find it to be quite refreshing.

Wheatgrass can be easily grown at home by planting seeds readily available online. I found my seeds at my favorite and very popular online store, and they were then shipped from an outside source. I have also noticed small sprouted pots in the produce section of my local food market. Keep in mind, however, that when you purchase the wheatgrass already sprouted, the first cutting may have already taken place. Many ingest a liquid or juice form of wheatgrass, and you may have heard of the health benefits of wheatgrass shots. Juicing makes the nutrients easier to absorb and may allow for healthier quantities of those nutrients. Because of this, you may feel energized within thirty minutes drinking wheatgrass juice. In lieu of juicing, you can cut the grass and throw it into a blender when preparing a smoothie. When doing so, your beverage will bear an earthy tone, and some may find its bitterness to be unpleasant.

The harvest time seems crucial. You want to harvest the greens typically around one week after you germinate the seeds at what is called the jointing stage. This is considered the nutritional peak, where the amount of chlorophyll, vitamins, enzymes, and protein supply are the highest. Many believe that they need to grow it in direct sunlight, but this actually contributes to the bitterness. Instead, expose the grass only to indirect sunlight and harvest it right at the jointing stage when it is at its sweetest. One of the complications of growing wheatgrass is that it is easily contaminated with mold due to its tightly bound roots in moist soil. If this occurs and you ingest it, the mold can make you sick. This white-colored mold typically grows at the bottom of the wheatgrass near the soil. Keeping a gentle breeze blowing, keeping the humidity low, and reducing the quantity of seed so the growth is less dense are three approaches to help limit this occurrence.

Things to Avoid

Omega-6 Fatty Acids

Considered necessary for human health, essential fatty acids can only be acquired from food; the body cannot produce them otherwise. The American Health Foundation theorizes that "omega-6 fats contribute to the metastasis and spread of cancer."[73] While omega-3 fatty acids reduce inflammation, most omega-6 fatty acids tend to promote inflammation. Anything that drives inflammation should be considered an adversary to cancer prevention. These polyunsaturated fats can be found in most vegetable oils, margarines, processed foods, and fried foods. Now, more than ever, doctors are beginning to discover the potential perils that accompany the overuse of omega-6 fatty acids. Our Western diet now contains as much as twenty times more omega-6 fats as omega-3 fats, leading to an unhealthy ratio. "The typical American diet tends to contain 14 - 25 times more omega-6 fatty acids than omega-3 fatty acids."[74] With excessive amounts of omega-6 being consumed, this ratio seems critical. The ideal ratio should be something closer to 1:1.

Another problem with a high omega-6 intake is the fact that the "double bonds within the fatty acid molecules decrease its stability and increase the likelihood of oxidative reactions. Because omega-6 poly-unsaturated fats are much less stable and far more reactive, particularly to oxygen, they can quickly go rancid."[75] "They tend to react with oxygen, forming chain reactions of free radicals that can cause damage to molecules in cells, which is one of the mechanisms behind aging and the onset of cancer."[76]

What you can do: Substitute coconut oil, olive oil, or even small amounts of butter for the following: safflower oil, corn oil, soybean oil, peanut oil, cottonseed oil, grapeseed oil, borage oil, primrose oil, and sesame oil. Foods also made with omega-6 fatty acids are mayonnaise, commercial salad dressings, and nut butters.

Fats in General

The link between fat intake and cancer has been under discussion for more than twenty years. Most studies to date have shown little or no link between a high-fat diet in adulthood and an increased risk of breast cancer. However, there is discussion regarding how "eating a high-fat diet during the teenage years may play a role."[77] The type of fat rather than the total amount of fat may be important. In general, the definition of fat includes oils, butter, and margarine, as well as the fat in processed foods, meats, fish, and nuts. Some studies are indicating a link between high dietary fat intake and a higher risk of breast cancer. The *Journal of the National Cancer Institute* published a recent study that concluded a "high-fat diet increases breast cancer risk and, more notably, that high saturated fat intake increases risk of receptor-positive disease, suggesting saturated fat involvement in the origin of receptor-positive breast cancer."[78] High-fat foods tend to have higher amounts of calories, which can lead to excess weight—a detrimental factor in cancer avoidance. Also be mindful that estrogen is stored in body fat, so excess body fat means excess estrogen. Being overweight increases the rate of breast cancer in postmenopausal women.[79]

As we have eluded to, not all fats are created equal, and the main culprit of the bad news seems to lie with saturated fat. Saturated fats are found in meats, dairy products, and baked goods. Is it of any coincidence that these items have been already designated as potential contributors to cancer? Based on current evidence at hand, it appears that saturated fat does play a role in increasing breast cancer risk. So think twice about eating that cheese and crackers. Depending on your circumstance, awareness and moderation is likely to be significant.

What you can do: Read labels and avoid foods with high levels of saturated fat, including meat and dairy products. Healthy fats include avocado, coconut oil, and olive oil.

Sugar

You may have heard the statement, "Sugar feeds cancer." In reality, sugar (or glucose) is a fuel needed and fed to every cell in our bodies, not just cancer cells. Sugar may be derived from bad choices like candy and sweets, or it can, if needed, be produced by our bodies via the protein and fats we consume.

Too much sugar without enough protein, fat, and fiber to balance it out can cause our bodies to make too much insulin. Perhaps it is not the sugar, but rather the excess insulin that may be a problem for spurring cancer cell growth. "By promoting obesity and elevating insulin levels, high sugar intake may indirectly increase cancer risk. In Dr. Christine Horner's column titled 'Natural Secrets for Breast Health,' women with the highest insulin levels have a 283% higher incidence of breast cancer."[80]

Sugar consumption has tripled during the past fifty years.81 Fortunately, or unfortunately, sugar—or rather, sugar-rich foods—is so prevalent in our modern-day society that we are consuming much more than our bodies can assimilate. And the way it is laced (or hidden) in food, you may not even realize how much you are eating and the impact it's having on your major organs. We were never meant to eat such large amounts of poor-quality sustenance. This excess in consumption seems to lead to several health problems, particularly chronic ones like diabetes, hypertension, and cancer, including breast cancer. One study evaluated the association between sweet food consumption and breast density, which is one of the stronger risk factors for breast cancer. Their analyses have shown that "high consumption of sugar-sweetened beverages, just three per week, is associated with higher breast density among premenopausal women and that high consumption of sweets foods, like desserts, is also associated with higher density among postmenopausal women."[82]

I've heard it said that cancer cells are immortal—that is, they don't die off in an orderly way like healthy cells do. Scientists have studied this effect and may have discovered what tumor cells do to avoid cell death. In laboratory research at Duke University, "cancer cells appear to use a combination of sugar and specific proteins to keep growing when they should die. These cancer cells appear to use sugar at a high rate, in order to ignore cellular instructions to die off."[83]

Keep in mind that eating sugar can increase your risk of breast cancer in another way too. "It delivers a major blow to your immune system. Your immune system is your natural defense against such invaders as bacteria, viruses, and free radical cancer cells. Sugar has the capacity to negatively affect your body's defenses by 50 to 94 percent after high sugar intake."[84]

If you are consuming aspartame or NutraSweet as an alternative or are considering it as an alternative, think carefully. "Dr. Soffritti with The Cesare Maltoni Cancer Research Center of the European Ramazzini Foundation performed a study on sugar substitute consumption in rats. They found that after being fed the human equivalent of four to five bottles of diet soda a day, the rats developed high rates of lymphomas, leukemias, and other cancers. At the highest dose level, 25 percent of the female rats developed lymphomas and leukemias compared with just 8.7 percent of the controls."[85]

What you can do: Cut back on sugar-loaded foods such as candy, baked goods, sugary cereals, and sodas to reduce your cancer risk. Over time you will crave sugar less, making it seem almost too sweet when you do eat it. Use white sugar sparingly and try natural sweeteners temporarily, which tend to have a lower glycemic index. Examples of natural sugars include: agave nectar, coconut sugar, date sugar, honey, and maple syrup. Also avoid artificial sweeteners. Consider additional control of blood-glucose levels through diet, supplements, exercise, and meditation.

Alcohol

Although you may not want to hear this, take your fingers out of your ears and listen up, because it is crucial. The consumption of alcohol may be a leading dietary factor related to breast cancer. A number of large-scale studies have shown a link between alcohol consumption and breast cancer. Not only that, but it would seem that the higher the consumption, the higher the risk.

According to the World Health Organization, "one in five alcohol attributable deaths globally (21.6%) can be attributed to cancer."[86] Professor Paul Wallace, a professor at University College London, believes "there to be a great deal of evidence to suggest that alcohol increases the risk of getting breast cancer. He also believes that how much you drink over your lifetime is what increases the risk. Drinking alcohol per se does not mean you will get breast cancer, it means your risk of developing it will be increased. There are some theories as to why alcohol seems to be shown to increase a person's risk of developing breast cancer. One reason may simply be due to the sugar content. Professor Wallace says that the increased risk is almost certainly in part because alcohol breaks down into a substance called acetaldehyde, which can cause genetic mutations—a permanent change in the DNA sequence that makes up genes. This can trigger a response from the body leading to the development of cancerous cells."[87]

In premenopausal and postmenopausal women, alcohol is thought to increase the production of the female hormone oestrogen, a female steroid sex hormone that is secreted by the ovary and responsible for typical female sexual characteristics. One characteristic of a cancer cell is that it multiplies out of control, and in certain types of breast cancer, high circulating levels of oestrogen can make this more likely to happen.[88]

Alcohol can also alter the immune system and contribute to nutritional deficiencies by interrupting the body's natural cycle of food breakdown. "Alcohol inhibits the breakdown of nutrients into usable molecules by decreasing secretion of digestive enzymes from the pancreas."[89] Alcohol is known to affect nutrient absorption by damaging the lining of the gut and intestines. Even if/when nutrients are absorbed, alcohol can alter the body's ability to properly transport and store them.

"The National Cancer Institute website states more than 100 studies that have looked at the association between alcohol consumption and the risk of breast cancer in women. These studies have consistently found an increased risk of breast cancer associated with increasing alcohol intake."[90] The Million Women Study in the United Kingdom provided a slightly higher estimate of breast cancer risk at low to moderate levels of alcohol consumption: "Every 10 grams of alcohol consumed per day, approximately one standard drink, was associated with a 12 percent increase in the risk of breast cancer."[91]

What you can do: Limit your alcohol intake. In accordance with the government's lower risk guidelines, women should not regularly exceed two to three units of alcohol per day. This amount would be equal to one glass of beer, a medium glass of wine, or two shots of liquor. Men would be allowed two drinks per day.

Food Additives

I will never forget viewing the special featured scenes at the end of the movie *End of the Spear*. The movie features true events in 1956 when missionaries traveled deep into the jungles of Ecuador to attempt to evangelize clashing tribes, hoping to teach them the value of life. The added scene shows the real-life character and tribesman Mincayani when he is brought to the states and experiences an American grocery store for the first time. To say that he is awed would be an understatement. He is amazed that no money is exchanged or item bartered at the checkout. You simply give the cashier a little plastic card, and when they are done with it, they give it back.

Our society, the United States, has reached a point in which food, both healthy and unhealthy, is readily available. We peruse the grocery store shelves and buy whatever we fancy, without thinking that there could be inadequate testing and perhaps government loopholes that enable ingredients to be used that show strong links to cancer. In fact, our government allow certain substances in our food that have been outlawed in other countries. It is becoming more and more difficult to decipher when we are being exposed to potential or even known carcinogens. Currently, "the FDA allows manufacturers to add small amounts of cancer-causing substances to the food you eat."[92] So it would seem that not only are many of our foods unhealthy, but they are seemingly unsafe.

The Environmental Working Group (EWG) has released a consumer's guide designed to help the average consumer protect themselves from what they label as The Dirty Dozen Food Additives.[93]

1. Nitrites and Nitrates[93]

These ingredients can be found in processed (cured) meats like bacon, salami, and hot dogs. These chemicals are used to preserve (stop the growth of bacteria) and add flavoring; however, studies suggest an association with several types of cancer. These chemicals are also used in fertilizers and rodenticides (to kill rodents). This may be why it has also been detected in fruits and vegetables and baby food containing vegetables.[94] According to the EPA, these chemicals, when used in fertilizers, readily migrate from soil to groundwater.[95] Check your food labels carefully and avoid products that list sodium or potassium nitrates and nitrites on them.

2. Potassium Bromate[93]

This ingredient is used in dough to make it stronger and to assist with rise during baking. It is a powder produced by passing bromine into a solution of potassium hydroxide. "It is listed as a known carcinogen by the state of California, and the international cancer agency classifies it as a possible human carcinogen (IARC 1999; OEHHA 2014). It causes tumors at multiple sites in animals, is toxic to the kidneys and can cause DNA damage (IARC 1999). Baking converts most potassium bromate to non-carcinogenic potassium bromide, but research in the United Kingdom has shown that bromate residues are still detectable in finished bread in small but significant amounts."[93] The United Kingdom, the European Union, and Canada prohibit its use in food.

3. Propyl Paraben[93]

Although it is a natural substance found in many plants and some insects, it is manufactured synthetically as a preservative for use in cosmetics, pharmaceuticals, and food. This substance is particularly good at killing or preventing the growth of fungus. Studies show that "parabens can affect the body similarly to estrogens, altering gene expression, including those in breast cancer cells. Research has detected the presence of paraben esters in 99 percent of breast cancer tissues sampled."[96] Check product labels for *propyl paraben* and avoid those that contain it.

4. Buylated Hydroxyanisole[93] (BHA)

Amazingly, this food additive is defined by Wikipedia as an antioxidant. It is an ingredient in a wide variety of foods, including chips, baked goods, and preserved meats. It is used to slow the oxidation of the fats and oils in food, delaying rancidity. By hindering oxidation, this preservative makes the food taste better longer. At high doses, it causes cancer in rats, mice, and hamsters.[97] The European Union classifies BHA as an endocrine disruptor. The Office of Environmental Health Hazard Assessment of the state of California lists BHA under "Chemicals Known to the State to Cause Cancer or Reproductive Toxicity."[98] Check food labels for BHA and avoid those that contain it.

5. Butylated Hydroxytoluene[93] (BHT)

This ingredient is similar to the latter, as it is a synthetic antioxidant and also added to food to prevent spoilage. These two ingredients act synergistically and are often used together. At least one study has shown "developmental effects and thyroid changes in animals, suggesting that it may be able to disrupt endocrine signaling."[99] A cancer link to human life has not yet been shown; however, most products containing BHA and BHT may be criticized on other nutritional grounds. Check food labels and consider minimizing your exposure to these ingredients.

6. Propyl Gallate[93]

This is also an artificial food additive used to prevent oxidation in cosmetics, pharmaceuticals, and food. It is sometimes used in conjunction with BHA and BHT. "A causal link between this ingredient and cancer in humans has not been established, however, it has been shown to be a modulator of estrogen receptor activity."[100] Even though the FDA considers this food additive to be safe, in other countries it is either banned or in very limited use. Potential side effects include stomach and skin irritability, allergic reactions, and impacted breathing. It may also cause kidney and liver problems. Check food ingredient labels and avoid buying products that contain it.

7. Theobromine[93]

Formerly known as xantheose, this phytochemical compound is a bitter alkaloid of the cacao plant.[101] It can be found in chocolate products, tea leaves, and the cola nut.[102] It is what makes chocolate extremely poisonous to dogs, because they lack the ability to metabolize it as quickly as humans. The darker the chocolate and more pure the cocoa, the higher the amount of theobromine. Like caffeine, theobromine crosses the blood-brain barrier, and the two are sometimes confused with each other.

Both are stimulants and are metabolized by the liver. A study published in 1993 compared men with very low levels of theobromine intake to older men consuming 11 to 20 mg and more than 20 mg of theobromine per day. The men with the higher intake were found to be at increased risk of prostate cancer.[103] Were the results due to the increased intake of theobromine, or did their older age contribute? One of the issues that EWG has with theobromine is that "it was secretly approved as GRAS (general recognized as safe) without notifying or sharing safety data with the FDA."[104]

8. Flavors[93]

There seems to be some ambiguity with the term ". There are natural flavors, artificial flavors, and incidental additives, which means that the manufacturer does not have to disclose their presence on food labels. Most packaged foods include both artificial and natural flavors. Both types of flavors contain chemicals. The real distinction lies in the source of the chemicals. "Flavoring mixtures added to food are complex and can contain more than 100 distinct substances. Consumers may be surprised to learn that so-called 'natural flavors' can actually contain synthetic chemicals such as the solvent propylene glycol or the preservative BHA."[93] Read labels carefully. The difference between foods listed with artificial flavors and those with natural flavors is pretty narrow. *Natural* might not be so natural after all. The concern with the term *flavors* is the vagueness of the term, because food companies tend to not fully disclose the ingredients.

9. Artificial Colors[93]

These are used in commercial food production and in domestic cooking to influence the flavor perception of the food. These became prevalent during the industrial revolution as workers became more dependent on foods produced by others. Tainted foods became popular because they provided a cheap method to return food, when needed, to a seemingly appropriate appearance. Many of these color additives, such as red lead for cheese and copper arsenite for tea leaves, had never been tested for toxicity or adverse effects. Not only that, but many of these coloring agents were intended for textile dyeing, not foods.[105] "Artificial colors, or FD&C (Federal Food, Drug, and Cosmetic Act) colors, were mostly derived from coal tar, which is a carcinogen. Now they are synthesized from petroleum."[106]

"Over the years, many FD&C colors have been banned because of their harmful effects. And it is likely that more will be banned in the future. Some of the worst FD&C colors include: Green #3, Blue #1, Blue #2, and Yellow #6, which cause allergic reactions and cancer in lab animals. Red #3 is a carcinogen, which may interfere with nerve transmission in the brain and causes genetic damage. It is banned in cosmetics but allowed in food, and it's especially harmful to children. Yellow #5 causes allergic reactions in those sensitive to aspirin. It may be life-threatening. Citrus red #2 is a known carcinogen. The only allowed use of it is to color orange skins. So, if you use orange zest in some of your recipes, you may be ingesting carcinogens. Any color with *lake* after it means that aluminum has been added to the color to make it insoluble."[107] "In addition, food dyes are not pure chemicals, they can contain up to 10% of impurities that are in chemicals from which the dyes are made or developed in the manufacturing process so they may contain cancer-causing contaminants. Although U.S. Food and Drug Administration (FDA) has established legal limits of these cancer-causing substances in dyes, certain factors are not taken into account. Tolerances were based on 1990 dye usage and did not consider the increased risk that dyes have on children."[106] As a consumer, what you can do is read food labels carefully to avoid FD&C-certified colors and choose whole foods over processed foods whenever possible.

10. Diacetyl[93]

Perhaps you have heard that microwave popcorn is unhealthy. Diacetyl is an organic chemical compound, a yellow/green liquid, with an intense buttery flavor. It is also artificially produced in factories across the country. It can also be found in candy, chips, coffee, and e-cigarettes. "It is a chemical linked to hundreds of injuries and at least five deaths. Whether natural or synthetic, the chemical can destroy the respiratory system when inhaled. It attacks the bronchioles of the lung. As the body tries to heal, scar tissue builds and further restrict airways. The disease is called bronchiolitis obliterans and the damage is irreversible."[108] In 2007 several companies planned to change their recipes for their butter-flavored popcorn to remove diacetyl.[109] A link to cancer has not been found to date.

11. Phosphates[93]

"These are among the most common food additives, found in more than 20,000 products in the EWG's Food Scores database. They are used to leaven baked goods, reduce acid and improve moisture retention and tenderness in processed meats. They are frequently added to unhealthy highly processed foods, including fast foods. In people with chronic kidney disease, high phosphate levels in the body are associated with heart disease and death. In 2013, the European Food Safety Authority began a high-priority reevaluation of added phosphates in food, but the deadline for completion isn't until the end of 2018."[93] A 2009 study linked dietary phosphate to lung cancer in mice.[110] "Foods high in phosphate include soft drinks, fruit syrup beverages, chocolates, ice-cream, biscuits, cookies, cakes, tomato ketchup, mayonnaise, processed cheese and soft cheese spread, frozen pizzas, hot dogs. Many natural foods also contain relatively high amounts of phosphate including egg yolks, milk, nuts, peas, beans, lentils, corn, mushrooms, and oats."[111]

12. Aluminum Additives[93]

"Aluminum is the most abundant metal the Earth's crust. It can occur naturally in food, however, most people are exposed through food additives. It can accumulate and persist in the body, particularly in bone. Additives containing aluminum, such as sodium aluminum phosphate and sodium aluminum sulfate, are used as stabilizers in many processed foods. The concern of EWG is the widespread use of aluminum combined with animal studies showing the neurological effect on animals when exposed in the womb and during development."[93] A 2007 study measured "significantly higher levels of aluminum in the outer regions of breast tissue, a predominant area for tumor formation. The breast biopsies were obtained following mastectomies and were evaluated using graphite furnace atomic absorption spectrometry (GFAAS). Whether the differences of aluminum content in the outer regions versus the inner are related to the known higher incidence of tumors in that region was not ascertained."[112]

Nutritional Recommendations

As we look at breast cancer rates around the world and how they vary by culture, we cannot help but consider food as a credible criterion for variance. Just because cancer runs in a family, does not mean that genes are a critical component. There are many factors that play a role in cancer development, and more and more research points to food as one potential catalyst. It may be that you have more power than you ever realized, should you be willing to make a change. Every one of us needs food to survive; however, it would seem that nutrition is somewhat optional. We have such easy and immediate access to poor food quality that nutrition often takes a backseat to pleasure and convenience. If you wish to be cancer free, it is imperative that you take a look at all facets of consumption. For the sake of longevity, you have the ability to use food for good or for bad, as a driver to or inference with cancer growth. It would seem more than theory to say that your food choices work together to create health or disease.

The best chance of survival may lie in adopting a diet that has been shown to protect women from breast cancer. The regions bordering the Mediterranean Sea, for example, seem to have the lowest rates of chronic disease in the world.[113] The people of this region eat a high amount of vegetables with high fiber and nutrition as well as 30 percent healthy fat in the form of olive oil. In fact, the more local olive oil they consume, the lower the incidence of breast cancer. Their diet is filled with not only olive oil, but also leaves from lettuce, spinach, Swiss chard, and purslane.

Experiment with some green food! Purslane, for example, also known as duckweed or pigweed, is a nutritional powerhouse, and although "native to India and Persia, it has spread throughout the world as an edible plant and as a weed. Purslane grows just about anywhere from fertile garden soil to the poorest arid soils. A rock driveway is nirvana to purslane. Purslane has fleshy succulent leaves and stems with yellow flowers. They look like baby jade plants. The stems lay flat on the ground as they radiate from a single taproot sometimes forming large mats of leaves." "Purslane is low in calories, rich in omega-3 fatty acids, and an excellent source of vitamin A, C, and B complex. Steam it, sauté it, or add it to your salads, soups, and smoothies. In addition to succulent stems and leaves, its yellow flower buds are also edible. Purslane seeds, which appear like black tea granules, are often used to make herbal drinks."[114]

Asian fare has been shown to deliver the lowest breast cancer rates in the world.[115] In China, for example, roughly 14 percent of their calories are acquired from fat, versus 35 or 40 percent by Americans. They traditionally eat a plant-based diet low in animal fat and dairy while high in fiber. Both the Mediterranean and Asian diets tend to be low on the glycemic index scale. Asia is also home to people of highest longevity.[116]

There are so many diets being discussed at any given time: Atkins, South Pacific, and Paleo, to name a few. The latest studies and research seem to be pointing in the same general direction. Call it of any name you choose, but a plant-based diet seems to offer you the highest chance of a life without cancer. What this means is that your diet centers around the consumption of plant material with everything else being eaten in moderation. It means avoiding or limiting foods from any source that ever had a face or a mother, including dairy and eggs.

As we have discussed, when food shopping, you should be spending the bulk of your time in the produce section or outside walls. The center aisles will house the overly processed foods like flour, sugar, and extracted oils. These processed foods are more likely loaded with artificial additives and preservative, as well as sugar that may be detrimental to your health. Keep in mind that when it comes to produce section of the store, the more color in a vegetable, the better. Studies show that women who have higher levels of carotenoids in their bloodstream have a lower risk of developing breast cancer.[117] Some of the best foods to get your carotenoids from are:

- Tomatoes
- Kale
- Carrots
- Bell peppers (all colors)
- Spinach
- Papaya (but not from Hawaii, as these are GMO)
- Sweet potatoes
- Cabbage (all colors)

According to Pam Popper, ND, the executive director of the Wellness Forum and author of *Food over Medicine*, "A plant-based diet may seem restrictive when you first hear about it, but actually, it lets you do whatever you want to do with maximum amount of energy for all the years that you are on the planet. It's not what's being taken away. It's what you are getting."[118]

There are those who will be unwilling to change their diets for any reason. The satisfaction gained by poor-quality food is simply too high for them. There may be an addiction that they cannot or are unwilling to face. Food addiction can be quite powerful, especially when candida (yeast overgrowth) is involved.[119] In the end, it simply falls back to choice, and you can only choose for yourself. You cannot change another's thinking pattern. By changing your personal eating habits for the better, you can, however, hope to influence those around you. Just as a smile can be infectious, so can your good eating habits. It has never been more apparent that changing your food will change your life.

NOTES

Chapter 6

RECIPES

> We cannot direct the wind, but we
> can adjust the sails.
> —Anonymous

Are We Getting Good Nutrition?

I travel a great deal for my job. One morning, as I sat in a Perkins restaurant waiting for my eggs because they don't have gluten-free pancakes yet (boo), I glanced across the room. There sat a woman, probably in her twenties, eating alone. It would seem that she had not been taught good nutrition or simply didn't much care for it. In front of her were two bowls of ranch dressing. She was eating breaded chicken fingers and french fries for breakfast, but not before dipping, of course. Ironically, she was drinking a diet soda. And yes, she was overweight.

That old saying may be true, you are what you eat, and many Americans simply do not know how to eat right. They may just be falling back on what they were taught or perhaps what they feel is comfortable and easy. Many are misinformed. An awareness of proper food choice when combined with positive action can have a profound impact on your health. It can be the strategic difference between living with disease and living with longevity. To be honest, now that I am somewhat reformed, cooking with fresh food is just as easy as cooking with boxed or processed products, if not easier.

Yes, you have heard my confession ... I am reformed—maybe not 100 percent, but I make many good choices now. If truth be told, I have been just as guilty of bad eating as most. I was raised on poor nutrition. It is what I knew. I was raised on meat and potatoes (the latter usually boiled) and a canned vegetable (green beans and corn). It wasn't until I hosted a foreign exchange student from Vietnam that it became apparent to me just how poorly I was eating. In fact, she asked, "Where's the vegetables?" When it comes to good nutrition, the more color in the food, the better. An easy way to increase your intake of fruits and vegetables is by blending or juicing.

Juicing versus Smoothies

A great nutritional option that is easily digested would be a smoothie or homemade juice. This can be used as a midday snack, a breakfast alternative, or even a bedtime regimen. To get the best nutritional kick, it is recommended that you juice/blend immediately before consumption, as vital nutrients diminish over time. Juicing is done with a juicer that separates out the pulp or fiber. I use the Jack LaLanne juicer. Juicing is one of the best ways to consume high amounts of fruits and vegetables. Certain fruits and vegetables should not be juiced—for, example, bananas and avocado. These do not contain enough fluids and would be better blended into a smoothie. If you have access to organic produce and can afford it, this should be your first choice. Store-bought juice is generally not considered the best alternative. It may contain much more sugar, and keep in mind that nutrients deplete over time.

Some fruits and vegetables require peeling and seeding due to the toxicity and bitterness of the skins or seeds. For example: Peel oranges and grapefruits, leaving as much as the white part as you can tolerate. Also peel kiwi, papaya, and anything that has been waxed. For fruit or vegetables that I am going to peel, I tend to not worry so much if I cannot find an organic option. Skins tend to have a great deal of nutrients in or just below them, however, so I prefer to buy organic versus peeling apples and pears, for example. Remove the seed from apples, peaches, plums, and all other pitted fruits and vegetables.

Here is how to prepare the produce before juicing. If you are not skinning the fruit or vegetable, wash thoroughly.

1. Fruit like apples: Quarter and core to fit the juicer. Seeds can be removed.
2. Carrots: Cut of the ends; peeling is optional.
3. Most vegetables: Clean thoroughly. Waxed cucumbers should be peeled.
4. Fruits: Bananas and avocados are too low in water content to put through a juicer. Melons should be removed from the rind; otherwise, wash fruits thoroughly.
5. Greens: Lettuce, spinach, kale, and virtually anything green and leafy should be washed thoroughly.
6. Rhubarb: Only juice the stalks. The leaves are toxic!

Mix and match as you see fit. Have some fun with it.

You don't have to necessarily follow a recipe to make a smoothie. You can add a couple of fruits (banana, apple, blueberries, strawberries, orange, etc.), a tablespoon of ground seed (chia, hemp, flax, or sesame), add one or more vegetables (celery, cucumber, spinach, carrot, etc.), add a cup of liquid (almond milk, coconut milk, water, etc.), and if it is summertime, you can add ice. You can vary the liquid based on the thickness that you desire. Do you want to drink it or eat it with a spoon? I usually also add a bit of rice protein powder. Smoothie made easy:

1. Blend leafy greens and liquid base together.
2. Add fruits and blend again.
3. Add booster(s) and blend again.

Greens: 1 cup spinach, kale, Swiss chard, or powdered equivalent

Liquid base: 1 cup water, coconut water, nut milk, kefir, or yogurt

Ripe fruit: 1-1/2 cups banana, berries, mango, peach, pineapple, orange, grapes, apple, pear, or combination; using a frozen fruit will naturally thicken the result

Booster: Chia seed, hemp seed, flax meal, natural nut butter, avocado, wheat germ, wheatgrass, ginger, herbs, probiotics, or protein powder

For blending the smoothies, I use a Ninja blender. I can simply peel and or core the fruit or vegetable and quarter. The blender will do the rest. Much of the time I merely put in what I currently have around the house. Here is an example:

1 apple, cored and quartered
1 avocado, peeled and pitted
1 cup almond or soy milk
Ice

Fresh leaves of kale, spinach, or other greens (If I do not have fresh greens, I add a powdered form)

1 carrot, ends removed
1 tablespoon flaxseed, ground*

At the end I might add, fresh ginger paste, raw honey, macadamia nut oil, coconut oil, olive oil, and/or probiotics, digestive enzymes, protein powder, mint leaves, wheatgrass, barley grass juice extract, liquid tinctures like zinc, etc.

* Ground flaxseed goes rancid fairly quickly, and whole seed will simply pass through the body. Buy them whole then simply grind in coffee grinder before consuming.

Meal Planning

When planning your meals, consider using food closest to the source, such as fresh fruit and vegetables, and be sure to include color— the dark greens, reds, and oranges. Stay away from or completely eliminate the packaged and processed foods. Start reading labels and looking for minimum ingredients. If you cannot pronounce an ingredient, you may want to do some research online and find out exactly what it is. If you are making a dish or casserole that contains rice or pasta, try using less of those ingredients and more vegetables. Our farmland in the United States is not as nutrient rich as it once was, so it's time to consider how you are preparing your meals. Are you creating food that will nourish your body, or are you creating a meal that will simply diminish the hunger?

According to Dr. Henry Mallek, records show that our diet is more key to our longevity than we thought. What if someone came along and told you that if you ate the right amount of foods that are present in the supermarket, you could live to be 120 years old? In his book *The New Longevity Diet*, he recommends the following nutrients:[1]

Nucleotides: These perform a range of functions in your cells and are precursors for the cells' DNA, especially in the cells of our immune and digestive systems when we digest them. Significant levels can be found in protein-rich foods like fish, seafood, and beef and some high-fiber carbohydrates like legumes, baby corn, and asparagus.

Saponins: These help prevent age-related immune system decline. These also help lower cholesterol and prevent cancer. These are found in one hundred different plant families, in foods like beans and tomatoes. Tomatoes contain a saponin called tomatine.

Phytates: This is an antioxidant that controls the effects of iron, which in excess can lead to the development of harmful free radicals, a breeding ground for cancer. Sources of this nutrient include seeds of plants. One of the best choices is whole grains. Milling wheat and rice removes phytates.

Protease inhibitors: These nutrients, as well as substances induced by them, interact with the cells' DNA to regulate and stop the cells from malfunctioning. Cauliflower, spinach, peaches, and plums are good sources, as well as tubers like potatoes and sweet potatoes. Be careful, though, as this nutrient is affected by food preparation. Prolonged heating inactivates them.

Glutamin: This building block of protein helps muscles function properly and helps the immune system function properly. It also helps maintain the supply of specific antioxidants made in our bodies. This nutrient is found in protein-rich foods, such as beef, lamb, chicken breast, turkey, certain fish, and some seafood. There can be small amounts found in cheese and certain grains.

Exorphins (carnosine): This protects DNA. Two servings of chicken, turkey, lamb, or beef will boost your body's level of this nutrient.

Pyrroloquinoline quinine (POQ): Only discovered in 1979, POQ is particularly important because it helps compensate for age-related decreases in activity of certain critical enzymes. Because humans and most animals don't have the capacity to synthesize or make this nutrient, the sole source for getting it is food. Foods contain extremely small amounts of this nutrient, but a little goes a long way. It can be found in vegetables like green pepper, spinach, and carrots. Fruit choices include kiwi and papaya. Beverages like green tea are also a good source.

Arginine: This amino acid stimulates and releases two very important substances in the body affected by aging: human growth hormone and nitric oxide. To get this nutrient, it is good to eat protein-rich foods such as meat and fish. More sources include cereals, bagels, crackers, muffins, and other foods with wheat. Nuts and legumes are also high in arginine.

Inulin and Oligofructose: These change bacteria in the colon to produce short-chain fatty acids (SCFAs). SCFAs remain in the colon to increase the ability of the immune system's function, facilitate DNA repair, and protect proteins from aging. Jerusalem artichokes and dandelion greens are two of the limited food sources. If you know how to procure Jerusalem artichokes, please let me know. Finding the other source, well, that shouldn't be a problem.

Taurine: This amino acid is found in practically every cell in the body with high levels in the brain. It is critical for heart functions, but levels decrease with age. This is important for the functioning of the body's metabolism and age prevention. Found in proteins, dark poultry meat has more. Shellfish (oysters, clams, mussels, and scallops) contain much higher amounts than shrimp, and the levels in white fish are about four times higher than tuna.

Lignans: Lignans modulate the body's hormone levels. Scientists have concluded lignans to have an antiestrogen effect. Unfortunately for those on a gluten-free diet, the best sources are barley and whole wheat. There is hope, though, for those with gluten allergies, because flaxseed contains the highest levels. Other sources include many beans, cowpeas, peanuts, sunflower seeds, and pumpkin seeds.

Quercetin: A strong antioxidant, this flavonoid also gives other antioxidants the opportunity to be as powerful as possible, getting rid of any cells that may be aged or malignant. Sources vary around the world. In Japan, tea is the principal source, while in Italy it is red wine. In the United States it is onions and apples.

Isoflavonoids Genistein and Daidzein: Isoflavonoids behave as estrogens and antiestrogens at the same time. Interestingly, they stimulate the body like a hormone, yet decrease the incidence of diseases caused by high hormone levels. Genistein plays many roles in preventing cells from growing too much. These nutrients are mainly found in soybeans. In Japan, where consumption is higher, woman experience a lower incidence of breast cancer. The latest research recommends consumption of only fermented soy products.

Isothiocyanates (toxin zappers): This nutrient, a key topic of this book, comes from a food family called cruciferous vegetables, which includes broccoli, cabbage, collards, and Brussels sprouts. They work against harmful chemicals and protect delicate tissue and organs like the breast from damage by xenobiotics (xenohormones).

Carnitine: The main role of carnitine is the transportation of fat into the mitochondria to supply energy. This nutrient is present in various foods at various levels. Particularly soothing to me is the fact that it is present at a rate eight times higher in ice cream than in butter. Beef has more than chicken. In general, fruits and vegetables have lower amounts than meats, chicken, and fish.

Phytosterols: These are the plant version of cholesterol. They interact with cells that line our blood vessels, preventing blood clots and preventing hardening of the artery wall. They also help prevent colon cancer by blocking the absorption of bad cholesterol, curbing the growth of harmful bacteria, and interacting with DNA to prevent gene abnormalities. This nutrient is widely distributed in vegetables. High amounts are found in Brussels sprouts, cauliflower, and okra. Peanuts, pecans, pine nuts, and pistachios are especially nutrient.

Glutathione: This nutrient is made up of three amino acids concentrated in the liver, lungs, and kidneys. These three organs, the toxic clearing house of our body, are brimming with glutathione to help get rid of unwanted chemicals. The older we get, the more glutathione we lose. This nutrient is found mainly in fruits and vegetables. Among the best fruit choices are peaches and melons. Among vegetables, squash, broccoli, and spinach provide excellent sources.

Recipes That May Contain Helpful Nutrients:

Omelet

6 eggs
2 tablespoons water
2 tablespoons miso mixed with 2 teaspoons water
2 mushrooms, diced
1 medium tomato, diced
1/2 red bell pepper, diced

Place eggs and 2 tablespoons water in bowl and whisk. Spray skillet with nonstick spray. Sauté mushrooms for one minute. Add eggs and stir until partially set. Place the miso liquid, tomatoes, and alfalfa sprouts in the middle of the eggs and spread in a long strip. Fold omelet over and cut into servings. Serve immediately.

Makes 3-4 servings. (Miso is made from the fermentation of soy.)

Fruit and Nut Muesli

> 1 cup rolled oats
> 2 tablespoons hemp seed
> 2 cups low-fat milk or milk substitute
> 2 teaspoons honey
> 1/4 teaspoon vanilla
> 1/2 teaspoon cinnamon
> 1/8 teaspoon nutmeg
> 2 cups raspberries, blueberries, or blackberries
> 1 small can mandarin oranges, drained
> 3 tablespoons chopped almonds, pecans, or walnuts
> 3 tablespoons raisins
> Pinch of salt

In a small bowl, combine the rolled oats, 2 cups milk, honey, vanilla, salt, cinnamon, and nutmeg. Chill in refrigerator overnight. Then divide the mixture among 4 bowls. Place 1/4 of the berries, orange segments, and nuts on each serving. Serve with milk.

Warm Salad with Vegetables

> 1 tablespoon parsley, finely chopped
> 1 tablespoon chives, thinly sliced
> 1 tablespoon basil, finely chopped
> 1/4 cup green onion, thinly sliced
> 2 tablespoons extra-virgin olive oil
> 1/2 pound asparagus
> 1/2 pound small, dry white beans

1 cup baby corn
2 cups broccolini or broccoli
3 carrots, julienned
3 quarts water, plus water for soaking beans
1/4 pound snap peas, trimmed
8 baby zucchini, quartered and cut into 1-inch lengths

In large bowl, combine parsley, chives, basil, green onion, and the oil. Discard the bottom part of the asparagus by cutting away the stiff portion, about 2 inches. Cut the asparagus diagonally into 1/2-inch pieces. In a saucepan, cover the beans with water, soak for 1 hour, and then boil for 1 hour until tender. Let cool and drain the beans in a colander. In large saucepan, bring 3 quarts of water to a boil. Add the baby corn, broccolini, baby carrots, and asparagus tips and pieces. Cook the vegetables for 2 minutes and transfer them to a colander, reserving the boiling water. Drain the vegetables well and place with the herbs and scallions. Add salt and pepper to taste. An herbal-infused olive oil tossed in before serving adds a nice touch.

Stuffed Green Peppers

4 large bell peppers (any color)
2 teaspoons olive oil
1/2 cup onions, finely chopped
1/2 cup pepper, finely diced (tops)
1/2 cup sliced mushrooms
2 cups mashed potatoes
1/2 cup parsley, finely chopped
1/4 teaspoon salt
2 large tomatoes, peeled and chopped
2 cups tomato sauce

Preheat oven to 350 degrees. Slice tops from peppers, and then remove the seeds and interior spines. In a medium saucepan, cook peppers in boiling water for 5 minutes or until slightly tender. Turn upside down on a paper towel to drain and set aside. In a saucepan, heat the oil and cook the onions, diced pepper from tops, and mushrooms until soft. Add mashed potatoes, parsley, salt, and pepper. Stuff peppers with the potato mixture and place them in a baking dish. Combine tomatoes with tomato sauce and pour over peppers. Bake for about 15 minutes, covered. Uncover and bake 10 more minutes.

Veggie Lasagna

> 1 medium onion
> 3 small zucchini
> 8 ounces mushrooms, sliced
> 1 can diced tomatoes, Italian style
> 6 lasagna noodles
> 4 ounces pesto
> 4-8 ounces shredded mozzarella cheese or vegan substitute

While noodles are cooking, sauté vegetables in coconut oil, olive oil, or a combination of the two until soft. Season to taste with salt, pepper, and Italian seasoning. Stir in tomatoes. In an 8-by-8-inch pan, layer noodles. You will need to cut off 1/3 to make them fit. You will intermix the pieces to make the 3 layers of 3. Using a spoon, butter the noodles lightly with pesto, and then, using a slotted spoon, cover with 1/3 of the vegetable mixture. Repeat twice. Cover with mozzarella cheese and sprinkle with parmesan (optional) and more Italian seasoning. Bake at 350 degrees for 30 minutes.

Other Recipes of Significance

Turmeric Tea

The most natural way to make turmeric tea is to use peeled and sliced root (about 2 inches) and add a few cups of water. Bring it to a boil, let it simmer on the stove for about 30 minutes, and then cover and let it sit overnight. In the morning you can reheat and dilute as needed. Fresh turmeric is slightly bitter, and a tea made with just the one ingredient is not terribly tasty, so you will likely want to add ingredients like honey, ginger, and/or cinnamon. You could also mix it with another tea of choice, like chai, for example. If you use dried turmeric for your tea, you may want to pay attention to the water temperature, because boiling it will make it less bitter.

Turmeric Tea Using Powder

2 cups water or 1 cup water plus 1 cup milk of choice
1-2 inches fresh turmeric root, peeled, or 1-2 teaspoons turmeric powder
1 teaspoon cinnamon or 2-3 cinnamon sticks
1 teaspoon raw honey

1/4 teaspoon ginger root or 1-inch fresh ginger, peeled

Pinch of clove

Black pepper for curcumin absorption as pinch or peppercorn

Optional additives before serving:

1 teaspoon coconut oil

Freshly sliced citrus fruit and/or juice

Heat on stove for 10 minutes. Blend well and strain if using root, and then drink hot or cool.

I find turmeric to be more tolerable when cold. As cancer loves sugar, consider drinking without the honey if you can tolerate it. You can also add a tea bag to help with the taste, like lemongrass, for example. You can also make a turmeric paste, a thickened version, and store it in the refrigerator for convenience. If your pets have joint issues, you can add this to their dog food.

Anticancer Marinade

This recipe, developed by molecular biologist James Felton, PhD, and his colleagues at Lawrence Livermore National Laboratory in Livermore, California, keeps formation of heterocyclic amines (HCAs) to a minimum. The marinade is especially effective when used with chicken, although it can be used with other meats as well.

The following is enough for one chicken:

> 6 tablespoons olive oil
> 4 tablespoons cider vinegar
> 4 tablespoons lemon juice
> 1/2 cup packed brown sugar
> 3 tablespoons grainy mustard
> 3 medium garlic cloves, crushed
> 1-1/2 teaspoons salt

Mix all ingredients together in a bowl. Place the meat in a container that will allow marinade to cover. Soak for four hours, making sure that the meat remains covered. It is very tasty.

Bone Broth

One day after I tweeted the merits of bone broth, I received a response from someone stating, "It's also called stock." Well, is it? According to *The Joy of Cooking* cookbook, stock is to be simmered for four hours. Bone broth, on the other hand, is to be simmered much longer—anywhere from twelve to forty-eight hours, which breaks the bones down, releases nutrients and minerals, and makes nutrient-rich collagen, gelatin, and glucosamine easier to digest. When I make bone broth, I will use the Crock-pot and use a duration based on the type of meat. It is very nutritious and easy to make.

Place your meat bones, preferably organic, in the pot and add water to cover. If using beef bones, the preferred mix contains marrow bones and bones with a little meat on them, such as oxtail, short ribs, or knuckle bones.

Add approximately 2 tablespoons apple cider vinegar (helps leach nutrients). You can boost your broth by adding herbs and vegetables before simmering.

Simmer for a minimum of 12 hours. The longer you simmer, the better the flavor. Season to taste. In general, it is recommended that beef be simmered longer than chicken. Let cool and strain.

You can drink it plain or use it to make soup, pasta, or rice.

Note: The gelatin that you might find when the broth cools is the crème de la crème—the good stuff. Adding pigs feet will provide more gelatin if you are making chicken broth. If you refrigerate overnight, you can skim any fat off the surface before serving. The broth can be stored for up to 5 days in the refrigerator and up to 6 months in the freezer. Filtered water, organic meat bones, and vegetables are preferred. Bone broth contains gelatin, calcium, phosphate, magnesium, glucosamine, chondroitin, and other trace minerals.

Breakfast Bowl

Breakfast can be especially challenging for some. Many in our society have been taught that it is okay to reach for that donut or stack of pancakes. These foods may boost those feel-good chemicals like serotonin and dopamine, but the spike in blood sugar that follows makes them a poor choice for everyday consumption. This wholesome bowl basically consists of a grain and fresh vegetables of choice. It's fun to plan ahead or sometimes just throw in whatever is at hand. It's a great option for any meal of the day. Adding an egg makes for a satisfying breakfast. Here is an example.

> 1 cup turmeric grain
> 1/2 cup chopped broccoli or zucchini
> 1/2 carrot, sliced or shaved
> 2 mushrooms, sliced
> 1/4 cup onion, chopped
> 1 egg
> 1/2 avocado, sliced (optional)

Turmeric grain:

You can make this with brown rice (many options), quinoa, millet, or any combination and turmeric. This will make several servings.

> 1 cup rice
> 1/4 cup quinoa
> 3 cups water or bone broth
> 1 tablespoon turmeric

> Combine all ingredients and cook in rice cooker or steamer

To make the breakfast bowl you can use a ceramic pan or well-seasoned iron skillet. (I avoid Teflon.) Fry fresh veggies in coconut oil and/or olive oil, season, and add the previously cooked rice. When vegetables have softened close to your liking, add the egg. You can stir the egg in or not. You can season to your taste; in fact, you can season differently each day. The vegetable choice is optional, and if it suits you, add 1/2 sliced avocado before serving. (This is considered a healthy fat.)

Up to this point, we have discussed the merits of making healthy and 'clean' food choices. I have provided you with some recipes that you might find helpful in reaching your sustenance goals. Now I would like to share some personal care recipes that might also support your goals to live a healthier lifestyle, keeping in mind that what we put on our skin or bodies might be just as critical as what we consume.

Constipation Emancipation

Chronic constipation can be a miserable and dreadful occurrence. I have suffered from its devastation for many years. In fact, I can remember many years ago being denied my annual Pap exam by my gynecologist until I had endured an enema.

According to the American College of Gastroenterology, you may have chronic constipation if you've experienced some combination of the following symptoms for three months or more in the past year:[2]

- Fewer than three bowel movements a week
- Difficulty passing stools
- Straining
- Hard or lumpy stools
- Abdominal discomfort and bloating
- Feeling like your bowel is never completely empty
- Feeling like there is something blocking your bowel
- Manual maneuvering to stimulate the bowel

It's important to discuss all your symptoms with your health care provider.

Possible causes of constipation include:

- Diet
    o Lack of fiber
    o Lack of minerals
    o Lack of sufficient fluid intake
    o Excessive dairy intake
    o Food allergies/intolerances

- Hormone disruption
    o Menopause
    o Perimenopause

- Low thyroid function, hypothyroidism
- Low adrenal function
- Pills
    o Prescriptions
    o Vitamins
    o Antidepressants
    o Antacids
    o Estrogen blockers

- Chemotherapy

Recipe for relief:

1-2 capsules magnesium L-threonate, 667 mg

1 capsule probiotic, minimum 500 million microorganisms

2 tablets calcium, 333 mg each, with magnesium, zinc, and D3

1/2 - 1 teaspoon C-Salts powder, buffered, non-GMO and nonacidic vitamin C

1 tablespoon psyllium husk powder, consider orange flavored if hard to tolerate

Stir in or shake the C-salts and psyllium husk powder into 8-12 ounces of water. Use this mixture to take the supplements.

I partake of this regimen at bedtime. You may find that you don't need all elements of the recipe. One of more of these ingredients may work for you. You could start with just the psyllium, and then, if needed, add the C-salts, then the probiotic, and then the minerals. Magnesium and calcium can also relax muscles and therefore help with sleep.

Magnesium Lotion

It would seem that magnesium is better absorbed through the skin than through ingestion. You can find magnesium lotion online, or you can make your own. This recipe calls for magnesium flakes, which you should be able to find at your local health food store. The magnesium is much better absorbed from flakes than from Epsom salt.

Ingredients:

1/2 cup magnesium oil (1 cup magnesium chloride flakes + 3 tablespoons water)

1/4 cup oil of choice, such as coconut oil

3 tablespoons unrefined shea butter or cocoa butter

2 tablespoons beeswax or emulsifying wax

4-6 drops essential oil of choice (optional)

In a saucepan over low heat, melt the shea butter and beeswax together, and then add the coconut oil. When melted, remove from heat. Heat filtered water just hot enough to steam, and then add 3 tablespoons of it to the magnesium flakes and stir or shake in a covered jar until dissolved. Transfer the melted oils to a blender or use a hand blender to start blending the oils. Adding a drop at a time will help keep the oil from separating later. All the oils will blend best if they are about the same temperature. Add the magnesium oil to the blender too, very slowly, blending between additions. Blend until well mixed. You may place the mixture in the refrigerator for 15 minutes to thicken and then reblend. Pour the finished lotion into a glass jar with a lid.

Use 1/8 teaspoon for small children and babies and up to 1 teaspoon for adults (possibly more for pregnant women) once daily or as needed. Spread on thin-skinned areas. Store at room temperature for 2 months or store in refrigerator, taking out an ounce at a time as needed. Refrigerated, it lasts for 3-6 months.

Caution: Those with an allergy to latex should not use shea butter. Consider cocoa or mango butter instead of shea butter.

Deodorant

I prefer this to store-bought deodorants, because it does not have any unhealthy additives like aluminum. I also love that it allows me to still sweat without the odor. After all, we were made to sweat, right? Simply rub a small amount into the armpit area.

Just mix equal parts of these four things:

    Corn starch
    Baking soda
    Shea butter
    Coconut oil
    (Essential oil of your choice is optional)

Toothpaste

Introduced in 1997, Colgate claims that Colgate-Total is the "only toothpaste approved by the FDA to help fight plaque and gingivitis." It has likely done so by blasting the teeth and gums with triclosan. Research suggests that "triclosan could cause breast cancer, though the results were gleaned from exposure in mice. Triclosan's effects on the endocrine system, which delivers hormones throughout the body, are also increasingly thought to be harmful."[2]

Base Ingredients:

> Coconut oil: Wonderful natural antibacterial and antifungal that helps bind the ingredients together

> Baking soda: An alkaline substance containing minerals that enhance teeth whitening

Optional Ingredients:

> Stevia: This natural sweetener may make it more palatable

> Bentonite clay: This natural substance can absorb toxins, heavy metals, and impurities Diatomaceous earth (food grade): A naturally occurring, sedimentary rock powder that adds abrasion

> Calcium and magnesium powder: Can provide a good source of minerals that may also whiten

> Essential oils: Adds scent and refreshment

> Salt: A natural element that can add abrasion

Example recipe:

>   2-3 tablespoons baking soda
>   1/2 cup coconut oil
>   5 drops liquid stevia or one packet SweetLeaf
>   1 tablespoon diatomaceous earth or calcium powder
>   5-10 drops essential oil, your choice of flavor (optional)

Detox Bath

>   1/3 cup Epsom salt
>   1/3 cup sea salt
>   1/3 cup baking soda
>   2-1/2 teaspoons ground ginger
>   1 cup apple cider vinegar

Laundry Soap

>   1 bar soap (pure Castile, Ivory, Zote, or Fels-Naptha)
>   1 cup Arm & Hammer washing soda
>   1 cup Borax
>   Optional: Essential oil, oxygen booster

>   Or

>   1 bar Castile soap, grated
>   4 cups baking soda
>   3 cups washing soda

Grate or shave soap. Mix washing soda and Borax thoroughly and then stir in soap. Add 20 drops of your preferred essential oil. Use 1 to 3 tablespoons per load. Add 1 tablespoon of oxygen booster for those tough loads. You can use a blender or food processor to mix.

Shampoo

> 1 cup water
> 1/2 cup fresh sage
> 1/2 cup fresh basil leaf
> 2 sprigs fresh rosemary
> 2 tablespoon Castile soap
> 1/8 teaspoon Xanthan gum
> 1 teaspoon almond oil
> Essential oil

While boiling water on the stove, place herbs in a mason or canning jar. Carefully add the boiled water, cap, and then shake gently for about five minutes, infusing the water. Strain. Add the remaining ingredients to the liquid and mix gently. Add 5-10 drops of your desired essential oil and then funnel into a recycled shampoo bottle.[3]

NOTES

Chapter 7

BODY COMPOSITION: MAINTAINING A HEALTHY WEIGHT

> *Don't dig your grave with your knife and fork.*
> —*English Proverb*

Obesity is quickly overtaking tobacco as the leading preventable cause of cancer. According to the National Cancer Institute, "Obesity is associated with increased risks of cancers of the esophagus, breast (postmenopausal), endometrium (the lining of the uterus), colon and rectum, kidney, pancreas, thyroid, gallbladder, and possibly other cancer types."[1] Obesity is "also linked to poorer cancer outcomes, including increased risk of recurrence and of both cancer-specific and overall mortality."[2] It has been estimated that continuation of existing trends in "obesity will lead to about 500,000 additional cases of cancer in the United States by 2030."[3]

In terms of breast cancer, "the stage of life in which a woman gains weight and becomes obese may affect the relationship between obesity and the cancer. Those who study this type of epidemic are actively working to address this issue. Weight gain during adult life, most often from about age 18 to between the ages of 50 and 60, has been consistently associated with risk of breast cancer after menopause.

"The increased risk of postmenopausal breast cancer is thought to be due to increased levels of estrogen in obese women. After menopause, when the ovaries stop producing hormones, fat tissue becomes the most important source of estrogen. Because obese women have more fat tissue, their estrogen levels are higher, potentially leading to more rapid growth of estrogen-responsive breast tumors."[3]

According to the *Journal of American Medicine*, more than a third of Americans are currently obese—not overweight, obese.[4] Obesity is defined by the National Institute for Health as having a body mass index (BMI) of 30 or higher.[5] It is now considered a medical condition when excess body fat accumulates to the point that it may have a negative effect on your health. The BMI formula is designed to provide clues to whether you are overweight, underweight, or at a healthy weight for your specific height.

To calculate your personal BMI:

1. Weigh yourself to the nearest pound.
2. Measure your height in inches.
3. Take measurement number 2 and multiply it by itself.
4. Divide your weight by the answer to number 3.
5. Multiply the answer to number 4 by 703. If you used metric measurements, disregard this step.
6. The answer to number 5 is your body mass index, or BMI.

For example: For a person who is 5 feet, 6 inches and weighs 133 lbs.:

1. 133
2. 66
3. 66 x 66 = 4,356
4. 133 / 4,356 = 0.0305325987
5. 0.0305325987 x 703 = 21.46

This person has a BMI of 21.46 and would be considered a healthy weight.

Guidelines are as follows:[6]

< 18.5 = underweight
18.5 to 24.9 = healthy weight
25 to 29.9 = unhealthy weight
>30 = obese

If you take a look at federal statistics, the number of overweight Americans has just about doubled in the past twenty-five years.[7] Obesity seems to be on the rise in all segments of the population. With the easy availability of unhealthy options and large portions, there is a propensity for Americans to eat whatever they want and perhaps a lack of self-discipline to stop eating when they are no longer hungry.

Junk food is high in taste-active components like sugar, salt, and fat. Monosodium glutamate (MSG), a flavor enhancer, is also found in most of these foods. Although the Food and Drug Administration claimed MSG to be safe in 1959, many experts now disagree with their findings. "It is the same neurotransmitter that your brain, nervous system, eyes, pancreas and other organs use to initiate certain processes in your body."[8] Even the FDA now claims *"Abnormal function of glutamate receptors has been linked with certain neurological diseases, such as Alzheimer's disease and Huntington's chorea. Injections of glutamate in laboratory animals have resulted in damage to nerve cells in the brain.*"[9] Labeling of MSG is becoming better, but traditionally, MSG was hidden in ingredient labels like autolyzed yeast, making it more difficult for consumers to recognize and address. Many people are sensitive to MSG and will exhibit immediate negative reactions. It can "make your heart race, cause drowsiness, weakness, and cause headaches among other things."[10]

There is no doubt that these taste-active components and flavor enhancers are doing damage while making you feel satisfied. Some people seem to have no problem controlling what they eat and the amount therein. Others, however, repeatedly find themselves eating unhealthy foods, even when they have made a commitment to change their habits.

The truth is that these processed, convenient junk foods stimulate certain areas of the brain associated with reward. "Upon consumption of these foods, the brain releases feel-good chemicals like dopamine, creating a euphoric feeling of pleasure. It is natural to seek out behaviors that increase levels of these positive neurotransmitters. In fact, brain imagining (PET scans) shows that high-sugar and high-fat foods work just like heroin, opium, or morphine in the brain."[11] For those who seem more susceptible, it can lead to a full-blown addiction. Multiple studies in rats show that they can become physically addicted to junk food in the same way they become addicted to drugs of abuse.[12] A food craving is essentially your brain signaling for more dopamine because you are experiencing withdrawal symptoms. "Brain imaging also shows that obese people and drug addicts have lower numbers of dopamine receptors, making them more likely to crave things that boost dopamine."[13] If you find yourself eating and craving these addictive, poor-quality foods, you are may be addicted yourself.

Dr. Mark Hyman discusses food addiction in his blog of the same name:

> Remember the movie *Super-Size Me*, where Morgan Spurlock ate three super-sized meals from McDonald's every day? What struck me about that film was not that he gained 30 pounds or that his cholesterol went up, or even that he got a fatty liver. What was surprising was the portrait it painted of the addictive quality of the food he ate. At the beginning of the movie, when he ate his first super-sized meal, he threw it up, just like a teenager who drinks too much alcohol at his first party.
>
> By the end of the movie, he only felt "well" when he ate that junk food. The rest of the time he felt depressed, exhausted, anxious, and irritable and lost his sex drive, just like an addict or smoker withdrawing from his drug. The food was clearly addictive.[14]

So if you feel I have done a pretty good job of describing you and your eating habits, you are not alone. Acknowledging the issue and understanding the ramifications is the first step. If you continue to eat these addictive foods, you are intentionally choosing *not* to eat nutritious foods with antiaging compounds. Your body and bodily functions will suffer the effects. Your body behaves the best when it is fed the best.

It is never too late to fine-tune your diet. As you wean off the convenient, processed food, you will eventually notice a corresponding decrease in cravings. Be patient and gentle with yourself. You will likely notice changes in your mood and energy levels when you choose to fuel your body in the way nature intended by eating foods made *from* plants, not *in* plants (factories). There are processed foods on the market now more than ever, and if you are unable to read and understand an ingredient on a food label, you might just want to consider not eating it.

Emotional Eating

Eating to feed the feeling, and not the hunger, is emotional eating. According to Jane Jakubczak, a registered dietitian at the University of Maryland, "Instead of the physical symptom of hunger initiating the eating, an emotion triggers the eating."[15] Women are especially prone to emotional eating.

Signs of emotional eating:

1. Your hunger has occurred suddenly.
2. You experience an intense and immediate need to satisfy a craving.
3. You continue to eat even after you are full or no longer hungry.
4. You suffer from feelings of guilt after eating.

"When your hunger is emotionally driven, you are more likely to reach for your defined 'comfort food.' It may not be about the food at all. Potato chips are favored by 36% of people that feel bored; happy people tend towards foods like pizza and steak while sad people will reach for ice cream or cookies, 39% of the time."[16] Stress, sadness, anxiety, and other negative emotions are considered potential causes of emotional eating.

Using food as a coping strategy is simply a distraction that keeps you from seeing and addressing the underlying issue. Not only will emotional eating not alleviate the stress, it will likely cause weight gain.

Suggestions to curb emotional eating:

- Try to recognize true hunger: Sometimes when we think we are hungry, we are actually thirsty. Also, a craving for sweets, chips, or cookies soon after a meal is not about hunger. You have already eaten.
- Try to recognize food triggers: Keep a journal record to help identify patterns in emotional eating, including emotions and feelings when eating, what and how much was eaten, and feelings after eating.
- Find comfort elsewhere: Instead of grabbing chocolate, take a walk, call a friend, listen to music, read, or treat yourself to a movie. Try to distract yourself from the emotion.
- Try to manage stress in a healthy way: The goal is to lower stress with healthful strategies, including regular exercise, adequate rest, communion with friends and family, and meditation.
- Be mindful of your eating: Mindfulness is a way of paying focused attention without judgment. Try to pay attention to the sensations, feelings, and thoughts connected with the food and you eating it.
- Stop buying unhealthy foods: Avoid stocking the cupboard or refrigerator with high-calorie comfort foods. Learn to substitute healthful comfort foods: a bowl of broth-based soup or a cup of tea.
- Make a point to eat a healthy, balanced diet: Between meals, choose low-calorie snacks such as fresh fruit, veggie sticks, or yogurt.

Inflammation's Contribution to Weight

It is quite possible that certain foods are causing inflammation in your body, thereby adding or causing you to hold onto weight. Food sensitivities that you may not even be aware of can cause your body to hold onto weight. I know that if I gorge on corn chips in the evening, I will weigh a pound more the next morning. The added weight is not so much from added calories or quantity, as it is from the type of food or quality. It is interesting to note that in Dr. Peter J. D'Adamo's book, *Eat Right for Your Type*, he recommends that a person of O blood type, which I am, avoid corn due to its effect on the production of insulin.[17] You might also consider a book by nutritionist Lyn-Genet Recitas. My sister gained valuable insight from it. In *The Plan*, she recommends trying a very noninflammatory diet before adding foods one at a time. As you add a food, you weight yourself to determine if it is causing inflammation.

The Importance of Physical Activity

Exercise has many benefits. It not only burns calories, but it also increases your metabolism throughout the day. In other words, when you exercise regularly, not only do you burn more calories with movement versus sitting, you likely burn more calories when sitting.

A study published on physical activity and global health estimated that 5.3 million of the 57 million deaths worldwide in 2008 were due to physical inactivity.[18] "In addition to controlling weight, exercise reduces the risk of a heart disease, cancer, the development of high blood pressure and diabetes, helps maintain healthy bones, muscles, and joints while releasing endorphins which promote psychological well-being."[19]

"More than two dozen studies have shown that women who exercise have a 30 percent to 40 percent lower risk of breast cancer than their sedentary peers. The female hormone estrogen seems to play a key role. Women with high estrogen levels in their blood have increased risk for breast cancer. Since exercise lowers blood estrogen, it helps lower a woman's breast-cancer risk. Exercise also reduces other cancer-growth factors such as insulin."[20]

The CDC recommends that adults "engage in moderate-intensity physical activity for at least 30 minutes on five or more days of the week," or "engage in vigorous-intensity physical activity for at least 20 minutes on three or more days of the week."[21] Examples of moderate-intensity and vigorous-intensity physical activities can be found on the CDC Physical Activity Web site: www.cdc.gov/physicalactivity/basics.

So when is a good time to start? A limited number of cancer studies have tried to evaluate physical activity across the lifespan. Studies that examined physical activity across different time periods in life found that "increased recent past physical activity was related to a reduced postmenopausal breast cancer risk, whereas physical activity during adolescence and mid- adulthood was unassociated with risk."[22] So it would seem that there is no better time to start an exercise regimen than *now*, or yesterday for that matter. Fitness, or lack of it, becomes more important the older we get.

"In 2014, postmenopausal women who in the past four years had undertaken regular physical activity equivalent to at least four hours of walking per week had a lower risk for invasive breast cancer compared with women who exercised less during those four years, according to data published in Cancer Epidemiology, Biomarkers & Prevention, a journal of the American Association for Cancer Research."[23]

As said by Agnès Fournier, PhD, a researcher for the Centre for Research in Epidemiology and Population Health at the Institut Gustave Roussy in Villejuif, France, "Recreational physical activity, even of modest intensity, seemed to have a rapid impact on breast cancer risk. However, the decreased breast cancer risk we found associated with physical activity was attenuated when activity stopped. As a result, postmenopausal women who exercise should be encouraged to continue and those who do not exercise should consider starting because their risk of breast cancer may decrease rapidly."[24]

Before starting your exercise program, sit down and evaluate where you are now and where you would like to be. It might also be a good idea to consult with your doctor. If you are currently overweight and your goal is to lose weight, you may devise a different program than if you are average weight and sedentary or not. If you can get a buddy involved, it will help you to be successful. If they can't do a program with you, at least ask them to hold you accountable.

Your age may also play a factor in how you proceed. You can determine how to calculate your target heart rate and maximum heart rate and use that to monitor where you currently with your regimen and when you need to bump up your workout. Don't get discouraged. For me, I know that it takes about three months of a program before I feel really good. You will get there. (If it was easy, everyone would be doing it already.)

Here are five steps to get you started:

1. Benchmark your current fitness level. For example, how many sit-ups can you do?
2. Design a fitness program. What do you like to do? What days, what activities, how long, and what time of day? You may want to do different things different days.
3. Obtain any needed equipment.
4. Design a plan and put it on a calendar.
5. Get started. Start slowly so that you do not burn out and always listen to your body.

6. Monitor your progress. You may need to vary exercise so you don't get bored.

To calculate target heart rate (where you want to be to improve cardio health), use the following formula:[25]

1. Calculate maximum heart rate: 220 – age = X
2. Multiply X by 70 percent (0.70)

Example for forty-year-old: 220 – 40 = 180 x 0.70 = 126

In this example, the maximum heart rate for this person is 180 with a target of 126.

So as you see, based on the formula, your maximum and target rates slowly decline with age.

Try to maintain your target heart rate for twenty minutes, but don't go over your maximum.

Potential Exercise Modalities

Yoga. A great stress reducer, yoga is known to increase flexibility, muscle strength, and tone. It improves balance, respiration, energy, and vitality. It assists with weight reduction, while improving cardio and circulatory health. Yoga provides improved athletic performance and protection from injury. If you cannot find a beginner class in your area, there are websites that provide adequate instruction.

Rebounding. A rebounder is basically a mini trampoline. You can pick one up online for a reasonable cost or find a used one pretty cheap. Rebounding is thought to be the most effective movement therapy for increasing lymph flow and draining toxins from the body.

When I did a health retreat, this was one of my daily routines. Many natural health practitioners recommend daily rebounding as a gentle detox technique or weight-loss aid. Due to the up-down movement, lymphatic fluid is forced to flow and flush toxins.

Walking. "One hour of vigorous activity a day can cut the threat by a whopping 25 percent, suggests a recent study published in Cancer Epidemiology, Biomarkers & Prevention. Walking at a brisk pace—which is approximately 4.5 mph or a 13-minute mile pace— is considered vigorous activity by the standards used in the study of more than 73,000 postmenopausal women. If you are more inclined to take a leisurely stroll, you're still doing yourself a favor: an hour a day reduces risk by 14 percent."[26]

Bicycle Riding. "Biking or walking just half an hour a day reduces risk of cancer according to a Swedish report published in the British Journal of Cancer. Compared with those who mostly sit during their main work or occupation, men who sit half of the time or even less experienced a 20% lower risk of prostate cancer. The study, which looked at more than 40,000 Scandinavian men ages 45-79, found a direct relationship between the amount of time men spent cycling and the risk of being diagnosed with cancer and their cancer recovery rate."[27]

It is always a good idea to check in with your doctor before beginning an exercise routine.

Tips for increasing your activity levels:

- Use stairs rather than an elevator.
- Walk or bike to your destination.
- Walk around the block after dinner.
- Exercise at lunch with your family, friends, or colleagues.

- Wear a pedometer or fitness armband or download a phone app to record your daily steps. Begin with a target of ten thousand steps.
- Join a sports team.
- Use a stationary bike or do sit-ups, leg lifts, and push-ups while watching television.
- Park a little farther from your office, the store, or the library for a nice walk.
- When the weather is too poor to be outside, do some mall walking.

Perhaps it is time to stop thinking of exercise as a chore. The term *exercise* is considered by some to be a negative term. Instead, consider movement as a precursor to longevity and a more fulfilling life. Like they say, if you don't use it, you're going to lose it. And if you do manage to live to a ripe old age, what would you like your *quality* of life to be like? It need not be a chore. Simply choose an activity you enjoy or think you might enjoy—and just do it.

NOTES

Chapter 8

ENVIRONMENTAL FACTORS/AVOIDANCES

> *The world is a dangerous place, not because of those who do evil, but because of those who look on and do nothing.*
> —Albert Einstein

We live during a period of immense and sometimes intense environmental impact. Human beings, in their progressive quest to produce and consume, have introduced a great many chemicals into the environment. Some of these chemicals, like dioxin, are a by-product of industrial processes and become quite destructive when they enter the body and accumulate in body fat. Others we produce to make our lifestyles more luxurious or convenient. Unfortunately, we may not recognize the dangers of these products until a breakdown in human health has occurred. At times, we can be our own worst enemy. Are we unknowingly fashioning our own extinction?

An example of chemicals that are produced specifically for our convenience is plastic. I challenge you to do your weekly grocery shopping without obtaining a product packaged in some type of plastic. The companies that produce these products seem more concerned about revenue than the negative impact they may place on living species. In fact, they may not even be aware of the impact. Their goal is to make a product that will produce demand and convenience, at the maximum price point that a consumer will pay. Unless or until a health concern becomes evident, the product will continue to be packaged in the same manner, indefinitely. The number of plastic containers used in the packaging and distribution of food and beverages is unrestrained and astounding. Why? Because it is cheaper to produce than any other medium. But "plastic is formed from synthetic chemicals that leach into our food and beverages, acting like an estrogen to the body."[1]

Pesticides are substances produced to attract, seduce, and then destroy or mitigate any pest. The Chinese began using sulfur as a pesticide centuries ago to control mold and fungus. Organic options and plant extracts eventually became effective for controlling pests; however, the convenience of the mass-produced synthetic pesticides and herbicides that came later pushed the nonsynthetics aside. During the world wars, synthetic chemical production exploded. After the wars, herbicide production began. Consumers and most policy makers were not overly concerned about the potential health risks of the widespread use of these synthetic chemicals. "Glyphosate, or Roundup, the world's greatest selling herbicide, is now being linked to damaged gut flora, a cause of Celiac Disease."[2]

Our Savior?

Close to fifty years ago, the administration of Pres. Richard Nixon created the Environmental Protection Agency (EPA). The Clean

Air Act of 1970, the Clean Water Act of 1972, and the Pesticide Control Act of 1972 were important regulations enacted by this new institution. The EPA now manages more than a hundred programs that sustain multiple major laws. These programs can be broken down into six basic categories: air, pollution prevention, wastes and recycling, toxics and chemicals, water, and pesticides. Controversies are rampant regarding the functionality of this agency, and "even the Supreme Court confirms that the EPA has shirked some of its responsibilities."[3] If you are relying on the government to protect you, be cautious. It might just cost you your health and/or, ultimately, your life. As Frank Sonnenberg, author of *Follow Your Conscience*, has said, "Trust is like blood pressure. It's silent, vital to good health, and if abused it can be deadly."

The Bad Guys

"The chemicals that are known endocrine disruptors include diethylstilbestrol (the synthetic estrogen DES), dioxin and dioxin-like compounds, polychlorinated biphenyls (PCBs), DDT, and some other pesticides. Endocrine disruptors, at certain doses, can interfere with the endocrine system (all hormones) in mammals. These disruptions can cause cancerous tumors, birth defects, and other developmental disorders. Any system in the body controlled by hormones can be derailed by hormone disruptors."[4]

The following is a list of the twelve worst hormone disrupters, also known as the dirty dozen:[5]

1. BPA[5] (Bisphenol A) is a "chemical produced in large quantities for use primarily in the production of polycarbonate plastics and epoxy resins."[6] "BPA has been linked to everything from breast and others cancers to reproductive problems, obesity, early puberty and heart disease, and according to

government tests, 93 percent of Americans have BPA in their bodies!"[5] It has also been linked to miscarriages in women, erectile dysfunction in men, lowered IQ, ADHD, and obesity in young girls. Avoid plastics marked with a "PC," for polycarbonate, or recycling label #7, most especially when purchasing food for children. Not all of these plastics contain BPA, but many do. Avoid receipts when possible, as thermal paper is often coated with BPA. Be cautious, however: chemicals used to replace BPA, like BPS, "may have nearly the exact impact, hormone disruption, as BPA has on the human body," according to a study in the journal *Environmental Health Perspectives*.[7] So instead of choosing a plastic product labeled "BPA-free," choose glass. Buy fresh food instead of canned since many of these cans are BPA-lined.

2. Dioxin[5] is a known carcinogen. It is formed during many industrial processes when chlorine or bromine are burned in the presence of carbon and oxygen. Dioxins are basically released by human activity. We created them. The burning barrel in your backyard, should you have one, creates dioxins. We are exposed to them when we eat contaminated food, which is very difficult to avoid at this point. "Dioxins are very long-living, build up both in the food chain and then the body, are powerful carcinogens, and can also affect the immune and reproductive systems."[8] A July 2002 study shows dioxin to be related to increased incidence of breast cancer.[9] "Animal products, including meat, fish, milk, eggs and butter are the foods most likely to be contaminated. One way you can cut down on your exposure is to eat a vegan diet".[10]

3. Atrazine[5] is considered by some a "21st century DDT."[11] "Atrazine is a highly toxic herbicide and carcinogen widely used on the majority of corn crops in the United States, and consequently it's a pervasive drinking water contaminant."[5]

There are websites dedicated to saving amphibians like the frog due to overexposure to atrazine. Why? Because male frogs exposed to Atrazine have become feminized, producing eggs for reproduction. "It has been linked to breast tumors, delayed puberty and prostate inflammation in animals, and some research has linked it to prostate cancer in people. You can mitigate your exposure by buying organic produce and by getting a drinking water filter certified to remove atrazine."[5]

4. Phthalates[5] are a family of synthetic chemicals used in a wide variety of consumer products. A 2010 study performed in Northern Mexico concluded that exposure to these chemicals may increase your risk for breast cancer.[12] They are a group of chemicals used to soften and increase the flexibility of plastic and vinyl. "Phthalates are used in plastic food containers and children's toys (recycling label #3) among other things. Some personal care products like vaginal douches, lotions and creams may also contain phthalates, so read the labels and avoid products that simply list added 'fragrance,'" since this catch-all term sometimes means hidden phthalates."[5] These chemicals behave like estrogens and can "induce proliferation and invasiveness of hormone receptor negative breast cancer cells."[13]

5. Who doesn't love a good Fourth of July celebration? Perchlorate[5] is both a naturally occurring and man-made chemical used in the production of rocket fuel, missiles, fireworks, flares, and explosives, and it "contaminates much of our produce and milk,"[5] according to Environmental Working Group (EWG) and government test data. "When perchlorate gets into your body it competes with the nutrient iodine, which the thyroid gland needs to make thyroid hormones."[5] Some call the widespread incidence of iodine deficiency a silent epidemic. "Thyroid hormones are important to regulate metabolism in adults and are

critical for brain and organ development in infants and young children. There are several research studies that link iodine deficiency with cancer risk and some medical doctors are using iodine to actually improve cancer outcomes. Therefore, current iodine research is calling for the use of molecular iodine for all patients with breast cancer."[14] You can reduce the effect of perchlorate by making sure to get enough iodine in your diet or by supplementation. Foods richest in iodine include seaweed, seafood (shrimp, cod, sea bass, haddock, and perch), and iodized salt.

6. Fire retardants, known as polybrominated diphenyl ethers, or "PBDEs, have been found to contaminate the bodies of people and wildlife around the globe—even polar bears. These chemicals can imitate thyroid hormones in our bodies and disrupt their activity"[5] and are pervasive in your home. They cover your furniture, including mattresses and child seats. "Exposure can lead to lower IQ, among other significant health effects. In 1999, some Swedish scientists studying women's breast milk discovered something totally unexpected: the milk contained an endocrine-disrupting chemical found in fire retardants, and the levels had been doubling every five years since 1972!"[5] If general exposure were not bad enough, were these items to catch fire, they turn into an absolutely toxic soup. According to the HBO documentary "Toxic Hot Seat," California female fire fighters are six times more likely to get breast cancer.[15] It is difficult to avoid these toxic chemicals due to regulations and excessive use. You can consider using a vacuum cleaner with a HEPA filter, which may cut down on toxic-laden house dust; avoid reupholstering foam furniture; take care when replacing old carpet (the padding underneath may contain PBDEs). Consider buying leather, wool, or cotton when replacing household items and check to see if the foam filling has been treated chemically.

7. Lead[5] exposure is a "contributing factor in the breast cancer epidemic in Nigerian women."[16] Other metals may be involved as well. Laboratory studies have shown that "a number of metals including copper, cobalt, nickel, lead, mercury, methylmercury, tin, cadmium and chromium have estrogenic effects on human breast cancer cells."[17] It's well known that lead is toxic, but it may affect your body by disrupting your hormones. "Common sources of lead include household paint produced prior to 1978, toys or household items (antiques) painted before 1978, toys made and painted outside the US (prevalent), bullets, curtain weights, and fisher sinkers, paint sets and art supplies, and storage batteries."[18] You can try to keep your home clean and well maintained (dust often) if older than 1978. Crumbling old paint is a major source of lead exposure, so get rid of it carefully. Drinking water exposed to lead should be of great concern. A good water filter can reduce this exposure.

8. Arsenic[5] is controversial. It is a naturally occurring mineral found in soil, bedrock, and water. You may have it in your drinking water. "Arsenic messes with your hormones."[5] Whether it messes with them in a good way or bad way is under debate. "Specifically, it can interfere with normal hormone functioning in the glucocorticoid system that regulates how our bodies process sugars and carbohydrates. Disrupting the glucocorticoid system has been linked to weight gain/loss, protein wasting, immunosuppression, insulin resistance (which can lead to diabetes), osteoporosis, growth retardation and high blood pressure. Arsenic is known to cause skin, bladder and lung cancer."[5] Interestingly, however, a Chilean study found that high levels of arsenic in drinking water were associated with a surprising drop in breast cancer deaths after residents were inadvertently exposed to high levels.[19] If this study holds water, not only could arsenic's tainted image be reversed, but you also may

see clinical trials in the future with arsenic being used in the treatment of breast cancer.

9. Mercury[5] is a powerful neurotoxin and, at certain levels, can cause neurological issues, autoimmune disease, chronic illnesses and mental disorders."[20] "Mercury is known to bind directly to one particular hormone that regulates women's menstrual cycle and ovulation, interfering with normal signaling pathways."[5] If you enjoy eating seafood, "wild salmon, halibut, perch, mahi, cod, skipjack tuna, whitefish, and trout are better choices. Avoid swordfish, tuna (bigeye and ahi), and orange roughy."[21] In Sweden they have conducted a number of studies where people with preexisting neurological and health issues (chronic fatigue-type symptoms) had amalgams removed; 78 percent reported improvement in their health status.[22]

10. "Perfluorinated chemicals (PFOA), used to make non-stick cookware, are so widespread that 99 percent of Americans have these chemicals in their bodies and it does not breakdown in the environment—ever. Exposure has been linked to decreased sperm quality, low birth weight, kidney disease, thyroid disease and high cholesterol, among other health issues. Scientists are still figuring out how PFOA affects the human body, but animal studies have found that it can affect thyroid and sex hormone levels. Avoid non-stick pans as well as stain and water-resistant coatings on clothing, furniture and carpets."[5]

11. "Organophosphate pesticides, produced by the Nazis for chemical warfare, was later developed by American scientists to target the nervous system of insects. Despite many studies linking organophosphate exposure to effects on brain development, behavior and fertility, they are still among the more common pesticides in use today. A few of the many ways that organophosphates can affect the human body include interfering with the way testosterone

communicates with cells, lowering testosterone and altering thyroid hormone levels. Buy organic produce to avoid these pesticides."[5]

12. "Glycol Ethers are common in solvents like paint, cleaning products, brake fluid, and cosmetics. Studies of painters have linked exposure to certain glycol ethers to blood abnormalities and lower sperm counts. And children who were exposed to glycol ethers from paint in their bedrooms had substantially more asthma and allergies. Avoid products with ingredients such as 2-butoxyethanol (EGBE) and methoxydiglycol (DEGME)."[5]

Other Substances of Concern

"Parabens are a group of compounds widely used as antimicrobial preservatives in food, pharmaceutical and cosmetics products, including underarm deodorants. Measurable concentrations of six different parabens have been identified in biopsy samples from breast tumors."[23] Here's what's not certain: the level of chemical exposure that might pose a risk to human health.

The National Research Council in July 2014 reaffirmed that "styrene—the key chemical component of foam cups and other food service items—might cause cancer in people."[24] "Styrene is used as a starting material in the manufacture of a wide range of plastics: polystyrene foam, synthetic rubber, plastic food wrap, photographic film, car parts, PVC piping, insulated cups, plastic bottles, and spectacle lenses. Styrene is used in adhesives, inks, cooking utensils, floor waxes and polishes, copier paper and toner, decorating materials (varnishes, putty, and paints), metal cleaners, asphalt, petrol products and carpet backing. We are exposed to styrene in the general environment by emissions from vehicle exhausts, tobacco smoke, incinerators and industrial sites, and by vapors from plastic and plastic foam products (off-gassing)."[25]

"Formaldehyde, a known carcinogen, is found in household cleaners, cosmetics (nail varnish), personal care products (soaps, deodorants), plastic foams (cushion fillings, insulation), fabrics (leather, furnishings, clothing, tea bags), building products (plywood, particle board, flooring), decorating products (paints including nail polish, sealants, pigments) and furniture. Exposure to formaldehyde in the general environment comes from vehicle exhausts, smoke (tobacco, coal, wood), dust and vapors off-gassing (being released) from construction, insulation and interior decorating materials, fashion and furnishing fabrics."[25] Is it any coincidence that when I became ill in my thirties, I was living in a new house, working in a new building, and driving a new vehicle? Talk about toxic overload.

"Chloroform is a colorless liquid with a pleasant, nonirritating odor and a slightly sweet taste. It is classified by the Centers of Disease Control as a volatile organic compound and reasonably anticipated to be a human carcinogen."[26] "It is an ingredient in medicinal/pharmaceutical products such as cough syrups, liniments, mouthwashes and toothpastes, and in domestic cleaning products containing bleach. Because chloroform is widely distributed in air and water, we are exposed to it in air emissions from pulp/paper and chemicals and drugs manufacture, vehicle exhausts, tobacco smoke, burning of plastics, and evaporation from polluted waterways. We are also exposed through water sources such as tap water, showers, and swimming pools."[25]

"Alkylphenol ethoxylates (APEs) are used as surfactants to lower the surface tension of fluids so they can foam or penetrate solids. They are used in the manufacture of textiles and paper, and are found in paints, industrial detergents, pesticides, herbicides, plastics, insulating foams, cosmetics, nappies and sanitary towels (as wetting agents), shampoos, hair-color products, shaving gels and spermicides. Studies have linked APEs in waterways and aquatic sediments to altered reproduction, feminization, hermaphrodism, and lower survival rates in salmon and other fish."[27]

It is only by creating an awareness of these and other negative environmental issues partnered with a willingness to challenge the status quo that can we hope to build a better, healthier environment. It has been shown to be quite possible. The Greenhouse Vertical Farm in Central Florida produces pesticide-free products for local markets, restaurants, and Walt Disney World. The forty-eight-by-forty-eight-foot greenhouse can reliably produce 135,000 plants a year with 5 percent of the water used by an outdoor farm. Shown to be sustainable, we can hope for an expansion of this type of production methodology.

Personal Care Products

I've heard it said that the average women puts more than 150 chemicals on her body per day. My mother, for one, was never, that I can remember, without lipstick and polished nails. The cosmetics industry uses thousands of synthetic chemicals as ingredients—even those linked to cancer, infertility, and birth defects. Many of these ingredients are not tested for safety, because testing is voluntary and controlled by the manufacturers. With the skin being the largest organ in the body, it would be wise to consider potentially toxic product ingredients. This means taking careful inventory of the household and personal care products you are buying and using on a daily basis. Toxic overexposure undoubtedly plays a major role in cancer development, and recent studies are finally starting to shed light on the worst offenders.

The Campaign for Safe Cosmetics, a project of the Breast Cancer Fund, lists many chemicals of concern. They are as follows: "1,4-dioxane, benzophenone, butylated hydroxyanisole (BHA), Carbon black, coal tar, known carcinogens, Diethanolamine (DEA), Cancer-causing formaldehyde and formaldehyde-releasing preservatives, hydroquinone, heavy metals like lead, arsenic, and mercury, nitrosamines, octinoxate, polyacrylamide, PTFE (Teflon), p- phenylenediamine, parabens, phthalates, Resorcinol, Retinol, synthetic musks, titanium dioxide, toluene, triclosan. Many of these ingredients are banned in other countries like the European Union, for example."[28]

There are apps that you can install on your smartphone that you may find helpful when trying to circumvent the cosmetic aisle of your local department store. The application that I am currently using is called EWG's Healthy Living. The Environmental Working Group, the nation's most effective environmental health nonprofit organization, created the Skin Deep mobile app. It is designed to help you shop smarter. You simply use the phone to scan the UPC label on the product. The app will then display a rating for that product between 0 and 10 for hazardous ingredients, with 0 being optimum. For example, I scanned Maybelline's Dream Pure BB cream. It scored a 2, showing low concern in three categories: cancer, developmental/ reprotoxicity, and low allergy. The application claimed no hazardous ingredients in the product. When I scanned Olay Total Effects 7 in 1 Advanced Antiaging Body Lotion, it scored a moderate 6. It scored low for cancer and developmental/reprotoxicity concerns but high for allergy concerns. Potential hazardous ingredients listed were propylparaben and fragrance.

NOTES

Chapter 9

THE BENEFITS OF ESSENTIAL OILS

> *Those who contemplate the*
> *beauty of the earth find reserves*
> *of strength that will endure as*
> *long as life lasts.*
> *—Rachel Carson, Silent Spring*

In late winter of 2016, I took a solo trip to the Caribbean—a sabbatical of sorts. There was no elevator at this particular economy hotel, so several times a day I would traverse the winding and circular stairways to the top floor. There was thick greenery on either side of the outdoor stairway. On one particular evening I stopped in my tracks. As the sun was setting, there seemed a subtle change in the air. The relative humidity changed, and the air became heavier; there was a beautiful, yet delicate aroma. I looked around and found that right next to the stairs, on the downward side, was a tree with beautiful white blooms that seemed to reach out and kiss me. I'm not sure what it was, but the bloom had the appearance and scent of gardenia. It was heavenly. It made me feel good, serene, and at peace.

There is no substitute for the calm, peace, and serenity that can be found while communing with nature. It was Alfred Austin who said, "We come from the earth, we return to the earth, and in between, we garden." So what better place is there to look for healing than in nature, in our gardens?

The use of medicinal plants to enhance healing has been in practice since the dawn of time. "The oldest written evidence of medicinal plants' usage for preparation of drugs has been found on a Sumerian clay slab from Nagpur, approximately 5000 years old. It comprised 12 recipes for drug preparation referring to over 250 various plants, some of them alkaloid such as poppy, henbane, and mandrake."[1] For many centuries, mankind has tried to find medications to alleviate pain and cure different illnesses. For centuries, the healing properties of certain medicinal plants were recognized, documented, and communicated to the successive generations. The benefits realized by each generation could be passed on to the next, with almost contact tweaking. The continued seeking of optimal health remains a present-day goal that offers continual future opportunities.

The word *essential* as a biological term is defined as a part which the organism cannot live or reproduce without. So when we discuss essential oils in this context, we are referring to the oil of the plant. "This essence is basically what circulates through all the plant tissue, carrying nutrition to the cells while carrying waste products out. For those oils that can be applied to the skin for example, they seem to do the same tasks as they do while inside the plant. They permeate the cell walls of your skin to deliver nutrition and remove waste."[1]

Essential oils are generally extracted by distillation, often by using steam. Other processes include solvent extraction, resin tapping, and cold pressing. There are various methods of use for essential oils. The aroma of essential oils can be therapeutic, the oils can be applied topically, and some can even be taken internally.

When procuring essential oils, there are various brands available from various vendors. Real therapeutic-grade essential oils can promote restoration and provide balance to all of your bodily systems; however, synthetic oils cannot. To make sure that you are getting a healing product, look for the words "100% pure" in the description. The bottle that it comes in should be tinted dark to protect the product from sunlight, and a list of ingredients should be clearly shown on the label. Synthetic oils are marketed in clear bottles and do not show ingredients or, if they do, don't list the botanical name. And keep in mind that if the price seems too good to be true, it likely is of synthetic origin. When storing your essential oils, treat them like you would a medication and keep them out of reach of children. A locked box may be the way to go.

Aromatherapy

To gain the benefits of essential oil aromatherapy, get yourself a diffuser. As I type this, I am enjoying the essence of a proprietary blend called Peace from Edens Garden. An aroma lamp is another option; however, the heat given off by the candle may affect the essential oil's composition and therefore healing properties. The units and oils can be found all over the Internet. Some diffusers also have LED lighting of various colors; if not healing themselves, they let you know when the unit has turned off. Many units can be used as not just a diffuser, but also as a humidifier, ionizer, and nightlight. Releasing essential oil elements into the air is a method of air purification, while breathing the gentle vapors of the aromatic oils is helpful at promoting relaxation and healing. A few drops (one to three) of oil per cup of water should suffice.

For the condition of breast cancer, the following essential oils can be helpful for use as aromatherapy:

- Frankincense
- Sandalwood
- Lavender
- Arborvitae
- Rosemary
- Lemongrass
- Clove
- Basil
- Geranium
- Clary sage

Topical

Essential oils can be applied directly onto the skin where indicated. They can also be diluted with water for use in a rollerball bottle, can be diluted when mixed with a carrier oil, or can be added to any lotion whether store-bought or homemade. *It is always recommended that you do a skin test first to check for sensitivity.* Be sure not to touch in or around the eyes if there is oil on your hands. It is a good idea to test and use an essential oil on children in a diluted form.

There are various carrier oils that can be used, and you may find that you prefer one over the other. Fractionated coconut oil is a type of coconut oil that stays in liquid form. Some other oil options include castor, avocado, jojoba, grapeseed, hemp seed, argan, and borage. There are also others. The various price ranges of these carrier oils may be an indication of what you may wish to try. Carrier oils can be found in health food stores or online. Roller bottles and glass containers can easily be found in similar locations.

For sore muscles and joints, oils or diluted forms of oil, can be applied directly to the inflamed area. A good topical area for holistic application of essential oils is the bottoms of the feet. The larger pores of this area allow the oils to enter the bloodstream quickly, but the toughness of the skin will deter the possibility of irritation. Some essential oils will have a warming effect and might be nice for those prone to poor circulation and/or cold feet. Examples of warming oils include cinnamon, clove, lemongrass, oregano, and thyme. Peppermint, on the other hand, provides a cooling effect.

For another topical effect, you can add essential oils to your bath; for example, lavender at bedtime might be quite soothing. Essential oils are concentrated, pure oil, so a little goes a long way. You might start with one drop for the bath or topical mixture, and then add a drop at a time until it is to your liking. In my previous section of DIY recipes, essential oils can be used for therapeutic and or aromatic benefits. For example, a spearmint oil could be added to the toothpaste, and a lavender oil could be added to the magnesium lotion. It is also possible to create an oil for daily use that is a blend of oils, like perhaps frankincense and lavender.

For the condition of breast cancer, the following essential oils are recommended for topical use:[2]

- Frankincense
- Sandalwood
- Lavender
- Arborvitae
- Rosemary
- Lemongrass
- Clove basil
- Geranium
- Clary sage
- Citrus oils
- Rose

Ingestion

Some, but not all, essential oils are safe for consumption. Make sure that what you are using is indeed safe for consumption. It is imperative that you are certain to be using a high-quality, pure oil and not a synthetic. For this category of oil, there are various methods of consumption. One method of ingestion would be to simply place a drop or two into a purchased veggie capsule and then swallow the capsule. This way, you gain the benefits of the oil without having to taste it. You can purchase these empty capsules online and assemble them after filling.

Another method of ingestion would be by drinking after dilution with water. A typical ratio for drinking is 1 drop of oil per 4 ounces of water. Some essential oils like lemon, tangerine, or peppermint might be great in water.

Some essential oils, like those blends specifically formulated for digestive issues, can be taken under the tongue. Start with one drop, see how you feel in a few minutes, and then you can consider another drop if you feel that you need it. It is best to start slowly and cautiously. You may experience relief pretty quickly.

And finally, another method of ingestion could be with food. You may want to add the oil as the last step before serving a hot dish to ensure that the therapeutic benefits of the oil are not challenged by the heat. For example, you could add oregano oil to an Italian dish or lemon oil to a lemon chicken dish.

For the condition of breast cancer, the following essential oils can be considered for ingestion:

- Frankincense
- Sandalwood

- Rosemary
- Lemongrass
- Clove
- Geranium
- Clary sage

Keep in mind that certain essential oils should be avoided for those who are pregnant or breast-feeding. Examples to avoid from the above lists include basil, clary sage, lemongrass, rosemary, and thyme. If you are pregnant or breast-feeding, check with your doctor before starting use.

Something to consider would be the use of homemade cleaning products to replace chemicals in your home. Some oils are great at cleansing, while others can kill bacteria and mold. Lemon, loved for its light, clean scent, is a staple in many homemade cleaning recipes. Other oils used for cleaning include, tea tree, rosemary, wild orange, lavender, eucalyptus, peppermint, and cinnamon leaf.

Essential oils have the potential to positively affect your quality of life. They can ease issues with digestion, complexion, circulation, immune function, cleansing, emotional balancing, and much more. Do your research before beginning, and have some fun with it.

NOTES

Chapter 10

THE MIND-BODY CONNECTION

> *The world we have created is a product of our thinking; it cannot be changed without changing our thinking.*
> *—Albert Einstein*

Thoughts Become Things

There once was a man who decided to take a sabbatical to a remote monastery. It was in a beautiful location, perched in the hills near the Alps. One fine day when the weather was pleasantly warm, he ventured out. Finding a scenic location, he lay down a blanket, settled in, and began his daily meditation. After a bit of time, a monk who was traveling nearby stopped to say hello. The monk was curious about the traveler, and after a bit of deep discussion, he asked him directly, "Tell me, what is it that you wish for?"

175

The man took a deep breath and surveyed his surroundings, contemplating an answer. The monk asked again, "What is it that your heart is longing for?"

With a bit of pause, the man provided the monk with a list of things that he thought, once achieved, would make him happy. He voiced each one with articulation and emotion. He felt in his heart that if he could just get all of the things on the list and be successful financially, then he would find joy. The list included material things, the repair of a tattered relationship, and a new job.

The monk listened intently and then quietly asked him one additional simple, yet nagging question: "What if you choose joy first?"

Do we have it backward? In my younger days, I can remember thinking that happiness was somewhere in the future. Sometime, someday, somewhere, I would reach it … eventually. Author Gregg Braden calls this preoccupation destination addiction. Then in midlife, I was blessed to realize the fault in my thinking. If happiness were always in the future, I would never achieve it. If you really think about it, the future, as well as the past, are not tangible. The only thing that is real is this very moment. *Now* is all that matters. I chose to make joy relevant, real, and present. I chose to choose happiness now, and you can too.

I have heard it said that our minds produce more than sixty thousand thoughts each day. What do your thoughts say about you? I am of the belief that what we think affects our health. A dear friend of mine was diagnosed with breast cancer in 2011. She was a good person. She was generous, loving, and kind. She was also overly dramatic. She was someone given to excessive emotional performance or reaction. It was her nature. Some might label her a drama queen. These types of people are sensitive to those around them and how they feel that they are being treated. It may even be more about perception than reality. Whatever the reason for this type of thinking, I can't help but wonder if her thoughts may have contributed to her ill health.

What about the negative emotion of depression? Could it be that if you are depressed, you are stuck in the past? Or if you are anxious, you are worrying about the future? And perhaps, if you are at peace, you are living in the present moment. If you find yourself reliving or rethinking about a past traumatic event or person, *you are potentially doing yourself physical harm.* Please read that sentence again. *You are potentially doing yourself physical harm.* How do your negative thoughts about the past serve your highest good now? That's right. They don't. There is nothing good that can come of them. Science is now accepting the theory of a mind-body connection. Could it be that your thoughts are making you sick?

A 1998 study of law students in their first semester of studies showed optimism to be associated with better mood, higher numbers of helper T cells (cells that influence or control the activity of other cells of the immune system), and higher natural killer cell cytotoxicity (providing rapid responses to viral-infected cells and response to tumor formation).[1]

How are your thoughts affecting your health? Would you rank your thoughts as mostly positive or mostly negative? What would your friends say about your thoughts? What story are these thoughts telling you? That you're not good enough? That you're ugly? That you are not successful because you don't own the right car or live in the right house? That you're fat or unlovable? Thinking in this manner reflects your perceived societal beliefs about yourself. They are not your truth.

The first step in recovery is to acknowledge your thoughts and realize that negative thoughts are likely not factual. They are simply a product of past programming. Although they can be quite toxic, they can also be reversed. When you catch yourself having a negative thought, ask yourself, *Where did that come from? Was it learned?* Most often the answer is yes. That negative thought is like a broken record. Fortunately, it can be thrown away.

Our behavior or thoughts are based on our beliefs, and our beliefs are based on our experiences. Where do your thoughts come from? If you were raised in a household of negativity, you were likely taught an unhealthy thought pattern. In her book titled *Why People Don't Heal*, Caroline Myss, PhD, calls this influence the "Tribal Power."[2] She says, "In tracking the souls of some people with cancer, I have often seen that early in their lives, a figure of some significance—a parent or teacher perhaps, said something to them like 'You'll never be good enough' or 'You'll never amount to anything.' It may have taken only three seconds, yet those three seconds commanded the rest of the person's life."

Words matter. So for the sake of your physical health, consider walking away from harmful relationships and draw close to you those persons who cherish and respect you—those who make you feel good, calm, and happy.

Many people have had difficult, abusive pasts. Children often experience dysfunction in the home. Parents can make bad choices, acting and speaking to their children in a very toxic manner. That experience is hard on a child and can lead to the same pattern within themselves, later in life. Children are not aware that they are being negatively programmed, and they can't likely walk away from the relationship. So why do parents do it? Perhaps they had a difficult childhood themselves and are reliving their own painful, negative patterns of the past.

So how do you break the cycle? You simply stop thinking those thoughts. When you find yourself thinking them, replace the thought with a present-moment positive thought. It may be helpful to write it down. Simply write down the fear or negative thought, draw an arrow to the right, and then write an associated, positive counterthought. By reframing it, you give yourself permission to heal. Perhaps it's not your past that threatens your peace, but rather your perception of it.

My childhood was not the best. My parents divorced when I was in second grade, and we lived with my grandparents for a short time. When the divorce was final, we moved back to the same hometown, and my mother immediately married a neighbor. Events became progressively worse.

Like many people, my stepfather had issues. It was difficult to predict what would set him off, and I was constantly walking on eggshells. Let me be clear. He was verbally, emotionally, and physically abusive. He left me battered and bruised, inside and out. The only reprieve was when he was drinking. When he was intoxicated, he was happy and sweet. Unfortunately, that did could not happen often enough. His inner demons would always resurface.

On one occasion I was sitting on the living room floor, not far from the television. It was late one Saturday morning. I was in my early teens. Not feeling well, my throat was quite swollen and sore. I thought that if I made something hot and soothing, it might reduce the pain. So there I sat in my pajamas and robe, eating my Cream of Wheat, harming no one.

In he stormed, saw me sitting there, and immediately became angry. He was enraged. He had formed a story in his head. His story said that I was lazy and a noncontributor to the family unit. He would not tolerate such behavior. Without so much as a question as to my well-being, he took his massive hands (he was a carpenter) and wrapped them around my neck. While yelling excessively, he jerked my body completely off the floor, shook me, and then released his grip. I fell to the floor in a heap.

I began to hide. I wanted to be invisible. Only now am I able to truly see how my current triggers and emotions have been affected by my past. I chose relationships with people who were emotionally unavailable, people who easily dismissed me as a person. I chose relationships with people who made me feel the way I was already feeling (invisible).

This is one of many stories from my childhood. There are others. I tell you this story not to necessarily relive the pain. I tell you to encourage you to let go of the past. I have. I know that he was a broken man. His perception of the world was not the same as mine, and it is not my job to continue to carry his pain. He simply could not be healed. Perhaps it was the fact that he had lost a four-year-old daughter. She had tonsillitis, needed surgery, and did not survive. Could this be a prime example of not letting go of past hurts? What do we do with such tragedy? Would it have somehow helped him to reframe his thoughts? After all, his behavior was driven by his thoughts. His thoughts did not offer me much benefit, but how do you think they affected his health?

My mother could not fix him, of course, and she couldn't convince him to seek professional treatment. That can be a downfall of certain personalities. We think that we can fix people. We want very much to fix them, and we have good intentions, but it is of no use. Rescuing someone is a form of enabling that might not be beneficial to anyone involved. It has a self-serving objective to build our self-esteem and make us feel better (needed), and our best intentions to fix someone will not make it happen. A person must be willing to make the decision to fix themselves. First, though—and this is key—they must willing to take a look at themselves and admit that there is a problem.

The other issue at stake throughout that relationship was his pride. He was not willing to entertain the thought of asking for or receiving help. Why is it considered a negative personal trait to ask for help? Knowing that you have issues and wanting to better yourself is strength, not weakness. *Never be afraid to ask for help.*

When I graduated from high school, my mother took their son, and we left. We moved out and moved on. I found out about fifteen years later that he had terminal cancer. He was remarried by then with two more sons. I was planning a trip home to see family, and I called his wife to ask her if I could visit. I had no way of knowing that in just three days, he would pass on. The meeting was a healing time for both of us. I was able to simply release his old behavior, knowing it was not his true self. I left with the peace of knowing that I had indeed forgiven him. It was a gift of self-love. I had transcended my past and stepped, ever so gently, from darkness into the light. *Never be afraid to forgive.*

I want you to understand that I do not live with those past negative thoughts, and the reason I don't is because I simply *choose* not to. Marinating in your painful past memories and victim mentality will not heal you and will likely do nothing but cause harm. Many have had a painful past. The questions is, what have you done with it? Do you wallow in it, or do you use it for your greater good?

Adversity is like a strong wind: It tears away at our outer layers of existence to leave a sturdy resolve. We don't just go through tough times. We grow through them. And believe it or not, the choice to grow or not to grow is yours. There are lessons to be learned from every relationship, and sometimes, the lesson is in the letting go. *Never be afraid to let go.*

Even when it can be done, breaking off a relationship can be extremely difficult, especially when you think the other person will be deeply hurt. But keep this in mind: Sometimes the only way we can learn a lesson is through pain. Can light be seen without darkness? As hard as it may be, letting go might just be the best thing for you and a catalyst for not only your personal growth, but for theirs as well. Because not only do you deserve to be loved, you deserve to be loved in the way you *need* to be loved. *Never give someone the power to take away your joy.*

Wellness

How do you define wellness? According to Wikipedia, it is the freedom from disease. Maybe so, but that seems a bit limiting. That definition defines what it is not. The full definition of wellness is much more. It is filled with richness and beauty. I'm going to go out on a limb here and tell you that your wellness is not necessarily defined by your medical test results. Although they can be helpful, they are not all-encompassing or holistic. Might they be limited by the knowledge and thoroughness of the particular doctor who orders them?

Perhaps there are several facets of wellness. There is the physical wellness—your physical body parts and the aches and pains or lack thereof. This is the description most often used. Mental illness cannot be omitted. There is emotional wellness—the wounds and/or the blockages that may prevent you from rising to your full and most beautiful potential. For example, are you setting personal boundaries as needed, and are you keeping them? Love cannot exist without boundaries. Do your relationships contribute to your wellness, and if so, how? Is there a person in your life who is not serving your highest good? If you answer yes, give yourself permission to shift, heal, or discontinue that relationship. It is my opinion that a harmful relationship will indeed affect your physical health. You are the captain of your ship, and that means that at certain times in your life, you must steer yourself to calmer waters. If not you, then who?

Relationships are perhaps the greatest catalyst in our emotional and spiritual growth. What a different world it would be if we all took the doctor's oath: First do no harm. It should be everyone's personal mantra. The first time I can remember feeling a personal disconnect with a close friend was in junior high school. We had been very close friends since the third grade and spent a great deal of time together. It became apparent to me, however, that her behavior was insensitive. She had a competitive nature that brought about this negative need to attack. It felt hurtful. It felt wrong. It made me sad. It was the first time, and not the last, that I felt the call to self-love. It was indeed time to save myself and to sever the friendship. There are lessons, however, in every relationship. Even when bad, relationships can offer insight into self-awareness—that is, if one is willing to take a look and face the music. Self-discovery doesn't have to be painful. In fact, it can provide great opportunities for transformation.

After spending a great deal of time with someone, we may feel comfortable even in an unhealthy environment. There can be a reluctance to let go, even when we are abused or neglected in that relationship. It is not unusual to repeat negative patterns from childhood. The inner child may come forward to tell us that we do not deserve better, and/or it may project doubt that our decision is really not for our highest good. It is in those times when we must remember that our true nature is love. We must learn to give love and receive love unconditionally—to ourselves and to others. That does not mean that you need be a doormat. Seeing the God (good) in all others can sometimes distract us from a person's desire to do us harm, whether their actions be conscious or unconscious. If you find that someone is harmful to you, without remorse, simply remove yourself from their presence. Let them be. Have peace in knowing that we are each walking our own journey, and someone else's lessons are likely different than your own. It is not your job to teach them that lesson. They must learn it through their own self-discovery. It is in that space that we (they) find peace and healing.

My brother, a chemistry professor, explains it this way: In chemistry, an atom will seek the lowest energy state, and this process dictates how bonds function. Our emotional state is similar. Living in dysfunction is living in a low-energy state. It feels right on some level. In fact, how you are wired in childhood can become your low-energy state. So, continuing with the chemistry analogy, to go from a low-energy state to a higher-energy state, you must input energy. So it indeed takes work, or energy, to bring yourself up out of a low energetic emotional state. You may have to take small steps up the emotional scale, but believe me, it is doable.

For example, this same brother grew up experiencing panic attacks. Fear of anxiety caused him to avoid certain situations that he knew would bring it on. So he was, in essence, living in constant fear. To break the pattern, he needed to face the fear. Doing so required expending more energy in the short term, creating a crisis of anxiety that would break the cycle. He needed to acknowledge its presence, allow himself you feel it, and then try to determine the source. You may try asking yourself, "When do I first remember feeling this emotion? What was going on with my life? Who was I with?"

Mind-Body Connection

Doctors have pondered the connection between our mental and physical health for centuries. "Until the 1800s, most believed that emotions were linked to disease and advised patients to visit spas or seaside resorts when they were ill. Gradually emotions lost favor as other causes of illness, such as bacteria or toxins, emerged, and new treatments such as antibiotics cured illness after illness."[3]

According to Dr. Fabrizio Mancini, "optimists live longer."[4] He says, "Fortunately, many people are asking: Is there a better way to stay healthy? Is there a better way to get healthy? Isn't there something better out there? The answers are yes, yes, and yes. Once this concept sinks in, you'll want to make self-healing a continuing operating principle in your life. There are many simple lifestyle options that can help your body self-heal. For example, exercise is self-healing and even a 10-minute walk can make a positive impact on mental and physical health."

You might consider this linear process. Our thinking affects our emotions, which, in turn, affect our health. Your body responds to the way you think, feel, and act. Your body reacts the same to an event as it does to a thought that mimics the event. Again, this is often called the mind-body connection. When you are stressed, anxious, or upset, your body tries to tell you that something isn't right. For example, high blood pressure or a stomach ulcer might develop after a particularly stressful event, such as the death of a loved one. The following can be physical signs that your emotional health is out of balance:

- Unexplained fatigue
- Depression, hopelessness
- Headaches
- Changes in blood pressure
- Trouble falling or staying asleep
- Stomach issues
- Changes in heart rate
- Sexual issues
- Stiff neck, sore back

- Excessive sweating
- Changes in weight

Tips to Change Your Thinking

- Use positive affirmations daily
  - o Buy an affirmations calendar
  - o Write and post sticky notes with affirmations
  - o Buy cards with affirmations
  - o Listen to audio with affirmations
  - o Talk to yourself in the mirror
- Seek counsel
  - o With a friend
  - o With a professional
- Meditate
  - o Find positive guided audio
  - o Write and record your own and play it back
- Listen to uplifting music
  - o Listen to what makes you feel good
  - o Dance to it
- Foster relationships with positive people
  - o People are influenced by people; choose wisely
- Reduce Stress and get plenty of sleep
  - o Practice deep breathing
  - o Go for a walk; seek exercise
  - o Take a vacation, perhaps alone
- Forgive yourself/others

A Call to Self-Love

What does it mean to love yourself or to practice self-love? Were you taught that this is a bad thing, maybe even selfish? I know that feeling, and it's wrong. When the flight attendant tells you to put the oxygen mask on yourself before placing it on another, it is for good reason. You simply cannot take care of (love) others if you cannot take care of (love) yourself.

Self-love can look differently to different people. Being a people-pleaser, for example, is a call to self-love. As we have been discussing, when it comes to your health, the quality of your inner dialogue is crucial. Forgiveness is another avenue in the journey of self-love. Forgiveness can take many forms and can go in many directions. We can be hard on others, but we can be hardest on ourselves. Forgive yourself for any past behavior that you have deemed as inappropriate. We are taught to forgive others, but we are not taught to forgive ourselves—our most important relationship. It is likely that what you did was based on past programming—programming that may have been dysfunctional.

When Jesus was on the cross, he is said to have whispered, "Forgive them, Lord, for they know not what they do." Forgive yourself because you could not see the consequences of your actions at that time. Forgive yourself because you did what you did because you thought what you thought ... for a reason. It is all right to make mistakes. It is my opinion that we are here, experiencing life, for the purpose of personal expansion, and that cannot happen without contrast.

It is through our mistakes that we find personal growth, learning, and meaning. Mistakes may not even be mistakes but simply an unconscious choice to learn and grow. I don't know about you, but I surely don't want to miss out on that. I can appreciate mistakes as a stepping stone to learning and personal growth. In the past I was quite hard on myself, beating myself up for regrets or mistakes that I perceived I had made. When, in fact, they were not so much mistakes as choices that I made, which then provided opportunities for certain experiences. Be compassionate with yourself. There will always be another layer of your outer shell to be broken. It's called *life*, and *change* is the only permanent part of life.

Start keeping track of judgmental thoughts you have about yourself and others. Then take those thoughts and rewrite them in an opposite, positive manner. Put those positive thoughts on sticky notes and place them at various locations in your environment. Change your thoughts, and you just might change your life. Remember that joy is not tied to circumstance. Whatever is going on in your life, choose joy. In words of the late Wayne Dyer, "If you identify with a negative kind of inner dialogue, rest assured that ego has temporarily separated you from your sacred self."[6] Acceptance means never turning your back on yourself. Make the decision today to love and respect yourself and others. That decision can improve your health and your life.

I like what Kyle Gray, motivational speaker, has to say about taking care of ourselves: "The truth is that how we treat our body is how we treat our soul." How are you treating yourself? To love all parts of yourself, including your shadows, provides a doorway to infinite possibilities. It is the gateway to self-acceptance and empowerment. And as said by Christianne Northrup, MD, "Loving everything about yourself—even the unacceptable—is an act of personal power. It is the beginning of healing."

Life Purpose

Are you struggling to find your life purpose? Why are you here? Life purpose is not dedicated to only a chosen few, and it's not necessarily about your daily job. Everyone is special, everyone has merit, and everyone has purpose—yes, even you. In the words of a dear friend, "The beautiful light inside you is meant to be a beacon of hope to others. You are here for a very important reason." Your life purpose can be complex but is more likely a simple product of giving. What is it that moves your heart strings? What is your passion?

Here is an exercise that you may find helpful: How to find your Life Purpose in about 20 minutes.[7]

The more open you are to this process, the more successful you will be and the less time it will require.

1. Take out a blank sheet of paper or open a word processor where you can type.
2. Write at the top: *What is my true purpose in life?*
3. Write an answer—any answer that pops into your head. It does not have to be a complete sentence. A short phrase in fine.
4. Now simply repeat step 3 until it makes you cry. It may take many pages.

When you are overcome with emotion, you have found it. That's it. To some people this exercise will make perfect sense; to others it will seem utterly stupid. If you persist, you will find the answer that breaks you. As you progress, some answers may be similar or repeated. That's fine. After fifty to a hundred answers, you may get distracted and want to give up or even get irritated. Push past this feeling and continue. Some answers may emit emotion but not make you cry. Keep track of those. Put a star by them, because they may be part of the larger picture. Keep going. Do it alone and in a quiet place. If you find your mind is not in the right place when you sit for this exercise, put the paper away and pull it out later when your heart is open and you feel ready.

Here is an example of one's finished product: "To live consciously and courageously a life of compassion, to awaken Great Spirit within others, and to leave this world in peace."

After about twenty minutes, this is what I arrived at: "To live authentically, capturing the essence and beauty of life, spreading the loveliest parts of it to those I encounter, thereby bringing to them peace, love, and understanding."

I say that this was the result after twenty minutes, but I did not do what I have recommended to you. I arrived at a beautiful statement of mission. It certainly sounded good. Is this my life purpose or what I want to be my life purpose? Because after arriving at this proclamation, it did not emit the emotional response I was looking for, and I took pause. As beautiful and elegant as it may sound, it did not make me cry. The epiphany came a few weeks later when a major breakthrough occurred. As I sat with my coffee early one morning, I opened my computer to reread the introduction to this book. Upon reading the last sentence, not only did it make me cry, it made me sob. This is it. This is my life purpose, and I embrace it. Thank you for being a part of my passion. Now it's your turn!

Stress

There are numerous emotional and physical disorders that have been linked to stress, including "depression, anxiety, heart attacks, stroke, hypertension, immune system disturbances that increase susceptibility to infections, a host of viral linked disorders ranging from the common cold and herpes to AIDS and certain cancers, as well as autoimmune diseases like rheumatoid arthritis and multiple sclerosis. In addition, stress can have direct effect on the skin, the gastrointestinal system (GERD, peptic ulcer, irritable bowel syndrome, and ulcerative colitis) and can contribute to insomnia and degenerative neurological disorders like Parkinson's disease. In fact, it's hard to think of any disease in which stress cannot play an aggravating role or any part of the body that is not affected."[8]

I've heard it said that stress is an event that we bring upon ourselves. The severity is, perhaps, something that we can control based more upon *our* perception than the actual event.

A relationship can be a catalyst for stress. It was more than twenty years ago when I found myself drowning in a bad relationship. Living with someone who was possessive and controlling had created a persona in me. I no longer knew who I was. I had lost my identity. To someone who has never been in this type of situation, it may sound crazy. How can you give up your true self and live each day as if you have been hypnotized, following another's influence, almost like a cult? If you know someone currently in this situation, please do not judge. Simply nudge. Nudge them to find the true answers and longings of their heart. Throw them a lifeline and pray that they have the courage to grab it and hold on. They will thank you for it one day.

Usually when we are in the midst of a bad situation or relationship, we cannot see it clearly. It is only after we step out of it that we can understand the true nature, destruction, and hold that it had placed on us. Trust your feelings. If your head and your heart are battling it out, your feelings (heart) that connect with your true self should trump your analytical thought pattern (your head). Ask yourself, what would bring you peace?

So on a weekend when he was away on business, I called in family, packed up my things, and left. Even in the worst of circumstance, it was not easy. I spent many days wrestling with my guilt and shame. My counselor was quick to affirm that when we have done nothing wrong, guilt is a useless emotion. Of course, she was right, but yet, I struggled. We can be hardest on ourselves. Can you relate?

But one day he found me. Perhaps he had followed me home from my workplace. I'm not sure how it came to be, but there came a day when a knock on the door found me face-to-face with him once more. My fight-or-flight response kicked in. I had to flee. I moved away. Within months of relocating a few hours away, I was able to find solace and heal. I slowly crept out of the darkness and forged ahead, making a new life for myself. It was good to be alone and independent. It felt good. Even so, I found myself fighting various forms of sickness for about a year. I know that it was lingering feelings of guilt and shame that were poisoning my thinking. I did not seek new professional counsel when I moved—something I likely still needed. I have no doubt that there is a direct mind-body connection, and that my emotions were affecting my physical health. It took a while, but eventually I was able to change my thoughts and regain my emotional and physical health.

According to HeartMath Institute research, here are some facts about stress:

1. Your body can not differentiate between a big or little stressor. Regardless of the significance, stress affects the body in predictable ways.
2. Stress can make smart people do stupid things. Stress inhibits a small part of the brain, and you simply cannot function at your best.
3. People can become numb to their stress. Some have become so adapted to the daily pressures, irritations and annoyances of life that it starts to seem normal.
4. We can control how we respond to stress. We do not need to be victims to our own emotions, thoughts, and attitudes. We can choose a healthy reaction.
5. The best strategy is to handle stress in the moment. Unfortunately, when we put off going for our own inner balance, our bodies have already activated the stress response and it's our health that suffers.[9]

Apparent links between psychological stress and cancer could arise in several ways. For example, "People under stress may develop certain behaviors, such as smoking, overeating, or drinking alcohol, which increase a person's risk for cancer."[10]

Dr. Susan Silberstein speaks about the correlation between breast cancer and stress.

> She has said, "We ask patients, 'Why do you think you got sick?' Ninety-five percent of them say they knew exactly where the disease came from, stress. Stress triggers a whole cascade of physical effects that can result in cancer. Stress may even be the most potent cancer-causing factor. And stress that's perceived as inevitable or uncontrollable is particularly damaging." Dr. Silberstein has served as Executive Director of the BeatCancer.Org since she founded the organization in October of 1977, after the death of her young husband to cancer. For several years, Susan taught the psychology of health and disease in the Graduate Division of Counseling Psychology at Immaculata University.
>
> "What's needed," she said, "is a balance between the sympathetic nervous system (the adrenaline rush that produces the 'fight or flight' response) and the parasympathetic nervous system (the 'rest and digest' relaxation response)." The sympathetic nervous system is like the accelerator of a car, and the parasympathetic nervous system is like the brake. Both are necessary, for obvious reasons. But in the typical cancer patient, the "accelerator" is stuck to the floor, and the "brakes" are out.
>
> Stress management and stress reduction techniques are essential to restore the cancer patient's proper balance. Dr. Silberstein recommends changing the stress-inducing

environment—if not permanently, at least temporarily. She suggests a number of helpful ideas, such as exercise, biofeedback, hypnosis, meditation, yoga, massage, laughter, play, prayer, pets, support groups, and counseling. She affirms that healthy relationships and having a purpose in life are essential.

According to Dr. Silberstein, "[t]he kind of disease the patient has is less important than the kind of patient that has the disease![11]

"Over the past 20 years, mind-body medicine has provided evidence that psychological factors can play a major role in such illnesses as heart disease, and that mind-body techniques can aid in their treatment. Clinical trials have indicated mind-body therapies to be helpful in managing arthritis and other chronic pain conditions. There is also evidence they can help to improve psychological functioning and quality of life, and may help to ease symptoms of disease."[12]

A team of scientists in Finland has used a self-report tool to reveal the effects that different emotional states have on bodily sensations. In 2016 there were five experiments and more than seven hundred participants from Finland, Sweden, and Taiwan. In the five experiments, participants were shown two silhouettes of bodies alongside emotional words, stories, movies, or facial expressions. They were asked to color the bodily regions whose activity they felt increasing or decreasing while viewing each stimulus. "The study reports that emotions affect our behavior and physiological states during survival-salient events and pleasurable interactions. The researchers thereby concluded that emotional feelings are indeed associated with bodily sensations."[13]

HeartMath Institute's research also shows how emotions change our heart's rhythm patterns. "Positive emotions create coherent heart rhythms, which look like rolling hills—it's a smooth and ordered pattern. In contrast, negative emotions create chaotic, erratic patterns. Using a heart rhythm monitor, you can actually see your heart rhythms change in real time as you shift from stressful emotions like anger and anxiety to positive feelings like care and appreciation. Coherent heart rhythm patterns facilitate higher brain function, whereas negative emotions inhibit a person's ability to think clearly. Coherent heart rhythms also create a feeling of solidity and security."[14]

Choose Your Response

So it would seem that your chosen response to a situation or stimulus might provide a direct link to the outcome. How you *feel* (mind/heart) might indeed correlate to *bodily feelings*. So can we limit bodily harm by choosing our thoughts or choosing a healthy response to that situation or stimulus?

I can distinctly remember a specific situation in which I chose to pause my thinking (to not fly off the handle) and instead chose a response that would provide what I thought would be a positive outcome. We had recently moved into a new home. The dining room was freshly painted and decorated in neutral colors. There was a painted chair rail with beautiful striped wall paper hung below it. Our daughter was entertaining a friend. They were gluing Popsicle sticks together and then painting them with craft paint. The situation seemed pretty harmless. I later learned, however, that the blue paint was not flowing from the bottle in a sufficient manner to suit our daughter. She squeezed that bottle with all the might that a twelve-year-old could muster, and it was absolutely enough. That beautiful blue paint splattered *everywhere*. It was on the walls, on the carpet, and all over the girls. It was then that I heard her call for me.

I could not believe my eyes. Phew, what a sight. How could so much paint come from that little bottle? My mouth must have dropped to the floor. Luckily, I immediately recalled something that I had recently read in a Stephen Covey book. He suggested that you "consider the outcome before choosing your response."[15] What a remarkable opportunity to put his lesson into action. I took a deep breath and said very calmly to our daughter, "Please take Heidi into the bathroom and get yourselves cleaned up." Then I walked into another room and calmly called down to my mother in the basement, who was visiting at the time. I asked if she might be able to come help me with something. We grabbed every rag in the house and began scrubbing until eventually the room was pretty clean. Our daughter still remembers this event mostly because I did not freak out and start screaming at her. I will admit that it was my first thought. I simply chose not to act on it. What good would that have done? We would not have been able to think clearly and do what needed to be done: clean up the mess. And now, it is a laughable moment to recall the sight of those two girls, eyes wide, covered with blue paint.

So whatever the situation, you can choose your response. Here is a simple formula to help you remember to choose your response.

$$A + B = C$$

Affair + Behavior = Consequence

Affair is the occurrence or incident that occurs. This affair or event causes certain emotions within you that then create a reaction or behavior in you. These two things, when combined, have a direct impact on the result or consequence. You may have no control over an event or affair (A), but by choosing a specific response or *behavior* (B), you can have a direct impact on the outcome or *consequence* (C). It simply boils down to this: In the end, what kind of experience would you like to have? In the end, what really matters?

Attitude is also a key to personal joy and happiness. Your attitude will play a big part in how you are able to choose your thoughts. As Charles Swindoll says, "We have a choice every day regarding the attitude we will embrace for the day."

Attitudes

The longer I live, the more I realize the importance
of choosing the right attitude in life.
Attitude is more important than facts.
It is more important than your past;
more important than your education or financial situation;
more important than your circumstances, your successes,
or your failures;
more important than what other people think, say or do.
It is more important than your appearance, your giftedness,
or your skills.
It will make or break a company. It will cause a church to
soar or sink.
It will make the difference between a happy home or a
miserable home.
You have a choice each day regarding the attitude you will
embrace.

Life is like a violin.
You can focus on the broken strings that dangle,
or you can play your life's melody on the one that remains.
You cannot change the years that have passed,
nor can you change the daily tick of the clock.

You cannot change the pace of your march toward your death.

You cannot change the decisions or the reactions of other people.

And you certainly cannot change the inevitable.

Those are the strings that dangle!

What you can do is play on the one string that remains—your attitude.

I am convinced that life is 10 percent what happens to me and 90 percent how I react to it.

The same is true for you.

Charles Swindoll (Used with permission.)

NOTES

LET'S WRAP IT UP

I truly hope that you have found the information in this book to be helpful. Currently, each year, about 247,000 new cases of invasive breast cancer are expected to be diagnosed in women in the United States. That's about 675 times per day that a woman hears the words, "You have breast cancer."[1] And this number doesn't account for the men. If there is any way to reduce this number, we must make a valiant effort. We must do our best to provide and spread useful information to prevent abnormal cellular activity that can lead to a cancer diagnosis. This is a call to action. Cancer isn't just an opportunistic bodily invader; it becomes problematic when the body loses its ability to heal itself. After you read this book, I encourage you to share it with at least one other person. Let us prove that we can control our destiny because we are each the captain of our own ship, and wisdom is the power that inflates the sails. It may not be an easy journey, but remember, smooth seas do not make for skillful sailors.

I've heard it said that more than 30 percent of cancer deaths could be prevented by modifying or avoiding key risk factors. So in this case, one-third of 247,000 is about 83,000 lives that could be saved; that's about 225 per day. Would you like to be included in that statistic? Not everyone who is educated on avoidance of cancer risk factors will be willing to make the recommended lifestyle changes; however, if not given the education, there is a much smaller chance they will succeed at evasion.

We have discussed various screening methods. Apart from a physical breast exam, mammograms are the recommended method for detection. Most recent guidelines released by the American Cancer Society recommend all women to begin yearly exams at age forty-five with the potential to change to every other year at age fifty-five. The guidelines also say that women who want one every year after age fifty-five should be able to have them. Women can start screening as early as age forty if they want to, and screenings should continue for as long as a woman is in good health. I was surprised that recent recommendations claim that breast exams, either from a medical provider or self-exam, are no longer recommended. I will do them anyway.

The debate regarding the efficacy of the mammogram and the proper screening schedule will likely continue. Sometimes I think that there are no medical facts, just opinions … and opinions change. Anyway, the goal of the screening mammogram is to find cancer early, when treatment is more likely to be effective. If we can increase the odds of finding cancer early by adding other safe screening methods, why not do it? After all, there is considerable evidence that "medical X-rays, which include mammography, fluoroscopy and computed tomography (CT) scans are an important and *controllable* cause of breast cancer."[2] Evidence also suggests that "risk of breast cancer caused by exposure to mammography radiation may be greatly underestimated."[3]

It also seems that how you metabolize estrogen may be an important risk factor in establishing your risk of breast cancer. I was found to have an unhealthy ratio of good estrogen versus bad when my breasts were at their most unhealthy state—TH-4 grade thermography. My sister seems to have the same issue, and I would expect that if my mother would have been tested before she lost the battle, the same results would have been found. What is going on? Although we cannot be certain as to the root cause or trigger, there is no denying the proliferation of fake estrogens in our environment and sustenance.

Our bodies have an innate ability to heal themselves and fend off disease, but if the body becomes weakened by environmental toxins and lack of nutrient-dense food, it is at a disadvantage. Our hope lies in our ability to control what we can. We must do our best to control what we are exposed to and the nutrition that we choose to partake or avoid. Unfortunately, what we do not know might be what kills us.

I encourage you to fight the fight,
To be true to yourself and your needs,
To know when to be silent and when to speak out,
To believe that you can control your destiny,
And to love yourself, no matter the journey or outcome.

And finally, I'd like to leave you with a poem that I wrote about the journey we share, the journey called life …

The Journey of Life

Do you know where are you going?
Did you bring a map?
Did you plot out the course?
Did you download the app?

You wanted adventure,
And before you it lie.
Your fear shall be banished,
In the blink of an eye.

Your future will be better
Than the past you have seen.
You are the creator,

You'll receive what you dream.

So set a true course,
Your inner compass will guide.
Through great twists and great turns,
Hang on for the ride.

Your mind may play games,
Though experience you must.
When they battle each other,
It's your heart you must trust.

And when you get to the end,
Of this journey called life,
Your greatest moments,
Will have come via strife.

You will determine,
How you did in this life.
Did you accomplish your goals?
Did you conquer the strife?

Always safe and supported;
Mighty angels at your side,
To love and protect you,
With pride they will guide.

So know where you are going;
Have a plan in the works.
Then relax and let go
God will work out the quirks.

Enjoy this adventure we call life. You are not alone, for I walk beside you …

Namaste

Feel free to reach out on social media:

Twitter: Christine Austin @savingtatas
Facebook: Facebook.com/savingurtatas
Website: www.christinemarieaustin.com

NOTES

ENDNOTES

Introduction

1   U.S. Breast Cancer Statistics, June 23, 2016 from http://www.breastcancer.org/symptoms/understand_bc/statistics

2   Kim Quinlan, "Breast Cancer by the Numbers," *The Courier*, March 14, 2014, http://www.thecourier.com.au/story/2150853/breast-cancer-by-the-numbers/?cs=62.

Chapter 1

1   Crown Copyright. SMEB0210 Story Museum. www.storymuseum.org/uk

2   "Oldest evidence of breast cancer found in Egyptian skeleton," Reuters, March 24, 2015, http://in.reuters.com/article/egypt-antiquities-cancer-idINKBN0MK1ZW20150324.

3   Olson, James Stuart (2002). Bathsheba's breast: women, cancer & history. Baltimore: *The Johns Hopkins University Press.* pp. 9–13. ISBN 0-8018-6936-6.

4   Robert A. Aronowitz, *Unnatural History: Breast cancer and American Society* (Cambridge, UK: Cambridge University Press, 2007) 22–24.

5   Ibid., 22–24.

6   http://www.cancer.org/treatment/understandingyourdiagnosis/examsandtestdescriptions/mammogramsandotherbreastimagingprocedures/mammograms-and-other-breast-imaging-procedures- types-of-mammograms

7   A. Van Steen and R. Van Tiggelen, *Short History of Mammography: A Belgian Perspective*, JBR-BTR (2007) 151–153.

8   S. S. Epstein, D. Steinman, and S. LeVert. *The Breast Cancer Prevention Program* Edition 2. (New York: Macmillan, 1998).

9   Mette Kalager, Marvin Zelen, Frøydis Langmark, and Hans-Olov Adami, "Effect of Screening Mammography on Breast-Cancer Mortality

in Norway," *New England Journal of Medicine*, September 23, 2010, http://www.nejm.org/doi/full/10.1056/NEJMoa1000727.

[10] L. Yaghjyan, GA Colditz, LC Collins, et al, "Mammographic breast density and subsequent risk of breast cancer in postmenopausal women according to tumor characteristics." Journal of the National Cancer Institute 103(15):1179-89, 2011. http://ww5.komen.org/BreastCancer/LowerYourRiskReferences.html#sthash.AF7TbGkP.dpuf.

[11] N.F. Boyd et al, "Mammographic Density and the Risk and Detection of Breast Cancer," *New England Journal of Medicine*, 2007;356:227-36.

[12] M. Durning, "Breast Density Laws by State," July 6, 2015, http://www.diagnosticimaging.com/breast-imaging/breast-density-notification-laws-state- interactive-map.

[13] M. Lee, "Mi-Jung Lee: Why my mammogram didn't find the cancer," February 27, 2014, http://bc.ctvnews.ca/mi-jung-lee-why-my-mammogram-didn-t-find-the-cancer-1.1707795.

[14] Pisano, et al, *Diagnostic Performance of Digital versus Film Mammography for Breast-Cancer Screening.* NEJM 2005;353:1773

[15] K. Schilling, "Breast Screening Tools for Dense Breasts with Kathy Schilling," http://www.areyoudense.org/resources/breast-screening-tools-dense-breasts-dr-kathy-schilling/.

[16] www3.gehealthcare.com retrieved January 29, 2016.

[17] J. Mercola, "The Greatest Weapon Against Breast Cancer (Not Mammograms)," March 3, 2012, http://Articles.mercola.com/sites/articles/archive/2012/03/03experts-say-avoid- mammograms.aspx#_edn11.

[18] G. Kolata, "Vast Study Casts Doubts on Value of Mammograms," http://www.nytimes.com/2014/02/12/health/study-adds-new-doubts-about-value-of- mammograms.html?mwrsm=Facebook&_r=0.

[19] A. Miller, C. Wall, C. Baines, P. Sun, T. To, S. Narod, "Twenty-five year follow-up for breast cancer incidence and morality of the Canadian National Breast Screening Study: randomized screening trial," February 11, 2014, http://www.bmj.com/content/348/bmj.g366.

[20] S. Begley, "Could This Be the End of Cancer?" *Newsweek*, December 12, 2011, http://www.newsweek.com/could-be-end-cancer-65869.

[21] G. Kolata, "Vast Study Casts Doubts on Value of Mammograms," *New York Times*, http://www.nytimes.com/2014/02/12/health/study-adds-new-doubts-about-value-of- mammograms.html?mwrsm=Facebook&_r=0.

[22] D. Kotz, "4 Steps to take Now to lower your breast cancer risk," *US News and World Report*, September 3, 2009, http://health.usnews.com/

health-news/blogs/on-women/2009/09/03/4-steps-to-take-now-to-lower-your-breast-cancer-risk.

Chapter 2

1   J. Mercola, "Why mammography is NOT an effective breast cancer screen," December 4, 2008, http://articles.mercola.com/sites/articles/archive/2008/12/04/why-mammography-is-not-an-effective-breast-cancer-screen.aspx.

2   http://anti-agingcliniccpc.com/Services/Thermography.htm

3   http://thebreastthermographycenter.com/articles/Thermography-Special-Report.pdf

4   http://articles.mercola.com/sites/articles/archive/2009/10/10/Simple-Steps-to-Lower-Your-Breast-Cancer-Risk.aspx

5   http://www.thermascan.com/patients.html

6   http://www.adelphatherm.com/#!untitled/c1dyz

7   http://www.iact-org.org/articles/articles-second-look.html

8   http://www.iact-org.org/articles/articles-second-look.html

9   http://www.breastcancer.org/symptoms/testing/types/thermography

10 http://breastthermographyevaluation.com/

Chapter 3

1   Science Blog – "Estrogen Linked to Sperm Count, Male Fertility." Science Blog. Retrieved March 4, 2008.

2   LR Nelson and SE Bulun, "Estrogen production and action," *Journal of the American Academy of Dermatology*, September 2001, 45(3suppl):s116-24. Doi:10.1067/mjd.2001.117432. PMID11511861

3   L Berstein, RK Ross, "Endogenous Hormones Breast Cancer Risk," *Epidemiol Rev* 1993; 15:48-65.

4   https://en.wikipedia.org/wiki/Estrogen

5   RK Murray, DK Granner, PA Mayes, et al, *Harper's Biochemistry, Twenty-fourth Edition*, (Stamford, CT): Appleton & Lange, 1996).

6   http://science.naturalnews.com/1998/11258403

7   http://www.calgarynaturopathic.com/Services/EstrogenMetabolism.aspx

8   Y Rong, L Chen, T Zhu, Y Song, M Yu, Z Shan, A Sands, F Hu, and L Liu, "Egg consumption and risk of coronary heart disease and stroke: dose-response meta-analysis of prospective cohort studies," *British Medical Journal 2013;346:e8539.*

[9] P Muti, HL Bradlow, A Micheli, et al, "Estrogen metabolism and risk of breast cancer: A prospective study of the 2:16 hydroxyestrone ratio in premenopausal and postmenopausal women," *Epidemiology* 2000;11(6):63 5-40.

[10] EN Meilahn, B De Stavola, DS Allen, et al, "Do urinary estrogen metabolites predict breast cancer? Guernsey III cohort follow-up," *British Journal of Cancer* 1998:78: 1250-55.

[11] P Muti, L Bradlow, A Micheli, V Krogh, JL Freudenheim, H Scunemann, M Stanulla, J Yang, D Sepkovic, M Trevisan, and F Berrino, "Estrogen Metabolism and Risk of Breast Cancer: A Prospective Study of the 2:15α-Hydroxyestron Ration in Premenopausal and Postmenopausal Women," *Epidemiology* Vol.11, No.6 (November 2000), pp. 635-640 http://www.jstor.org/stable/3703815?seq=1#page_scan_tab_contents.

[12] http://www.breasthealthproject.com/EstrogenMetabolites.html

Chapter 4

[1] Carolyn M. Cover, S. Jean Hsieh, Susan H. Tran, Gunnell Hallden, Gloria S. Kim, Leonard F. Bjeldanes, and Gary L. Firestone, "Indole-3-carbinol Inhibits the Expression of Cyclin-dependent Kinase-6 and Induces a G1 Cell Cycle Arrest of Human Breast Cancer Cells Independent of Estrogen Receptor Signaling," *The Journal of Biological Chemistry*, February 13, 1998, 273, 3838-3847 http://www.jbc.org/content/273/7/3838.long.

[2] Ibid., 3838–47.

[3] http://blog.doctoroz.com/is-this-right-for-you/diindolylmethane-dim-is-this-right-for-you

[4] http://www.rxlist.com/calcium_d-glucarate-page3/supplements.htm#Interactions

[5] "Diindolylmethane" from WebMD, http://www.webmd.com.

[6] http://wholehealthchicago.com/2009/05/11/alpha-lipoic-acid/

[7] https://www.scribd.com/doc/300935911/sources-of-alpha-lipoic-acid

[8] http://www.ncbi.nlm.nih.gov/pmc/articles/PMC1470481/

[9] http://www.cancer.net/navigating-cancer-care/prevention-and-healthy-living/diet-and-   nutrition/expert-qa-vitamin-d-and-cancer-risk#. VSnDdgi3dwM.twitter

[10] KM Blackmore, M Lesosky, H Barnett, et al, "Vitamin D from dietary intake and sunlight exposure and the risk of hormone-receptor-defined breast cancer," *American Journal Epidemiology*, October 15, 2008, 168(8):915-924. doi: 10.1093/aje/kwn198

11 JA Pennington and SA Schoen, "Total Diet Study: Estimated Dietary intakes of Nutritional Elements," *Int J Vitam Nutr Res*, 1996; 66 (4):350-62 from http://www.ncbi.nlm.nih.gov/pubmed/8979164.

12 http://www.optimox.com/pics/Iodine/opt_Research_I.shtml Publications by Guy Abraham, MD, on Iodine references at Optimox.com

13 http://cancerres.aacrjournals.org/cgi/reprint/35/9/2332 Bernard A. Eskin et al, "Rat mammary gland atypia produced by iodine blockade with perchlorate," *Cancer Research*, 1975 Sep; 35(9):2332- http://cancerres.aacrjournals.org/cgi/reprint/35/9/2332.

14 http://cancerres.aacrjournals.org/cgi/reprint/46/2/877 "Dietary Iodine Deficiency as a Tumor Promoter and Carcinogen in Male F344/NCr Rats" Masato Ohshima and Jerrold M. Ward. Cancer Research 46, 877-883, February 1, 1986, http://cancerres.aacrjournals.org/content/46/2/877.full.pdf+html.

15 http://content.nejm.org/cgi/content/full/353/3/229 "Benign Breast Disease and the Risk of Breast Cancer," Lynn C. Hartmann, *New England Journal of Medicine* Volume 353;3:229-237 July 21, 2005, http://www.nejm.org/doi/full/10.1056/NEJMoa044383.

16 http://www.ncbi.nlm.nih.gov/pubmed/8221402 W.R. Ghent, B.A. Eskin, D.A. Low, and L.P. Hill, "Iodine replacement in fibrocystic disease of the breast." *Can J Surg* 1993; 36:453-460 http://www.ncbi.nlm.nih.gov/pubmed/8221402.

17 http://clinicaltrials.gov/ct/show/NCT00237523?order=1 "Clinical Trial for Iodine treatment of Fibrocystic Breast Disease Study for Treatment of Moderate or Severe, Periodic, 'Cyclic,' Breast Pain." This study is ongoing, but not recruiting participants. Sponsored by: Symbollon Pharmaceuticals ClinicalTrials.gov Identifier: NCT00237523

18 S. Buist, "The Guide to Supplementing with Iodine" Rev 12/11 11 from http://jeffreydachmd.com/wp-content/uploads/2014/03/The-Guide-to-Supplementing-with- Iodine-Stephanie-Burst-ND.pdf.

19 Mark Sircus, "Iodine to the Rescue," June 11, 2012, http://drsircus.com/medicine/iodine/iodine-rescue.

20 Ibid.

21 http://www.westonaprice.org/health-topics/abcs-of-nutrition/magnificent-magnesium/?option=com_content&view=article&id=2303:magnificent-magnesium-croatian-translation&catid=135:croatian&Itemid=169

22   K. Czapp, "The Neglected Mineral We Cannot Live Without," September. 23, 2010, http://www.westonaprice.org/health-topics/abcs-of-nutrition/magnificent-magnesium/.

23   L.Euler, "The Doctor Who Cured Too Many Patients" http://www.cancerdefeated.com/the-doctor-who-cured-too-many-patients/1676/

24   http://www.westonaprice.org/

25   Kuljeet Kaur, Rajiv Gupta, Shubhini A. Saraf, and Shailendra K. Saraf, "Zinc: The Metal of Life," Vol.13, Issue 4 p.358-376, July 2014 from http://onlinelibrary.wiley.com/doi/10.1111/1541-4337.12067/abstract.

26   Cardiff University. "Zinc linked to breast cancer: Insight into body's zinc controls has implications for disease." *Science Daily*, February 6, 2012. http://www.sciencedaily.com/releases/2012/02/120206102954.htm

27   P. Holford, "The Truth about Vitamin C and Cancer," January 5, 2010, https://www.patrickholford.com/advice/the-truth-about-vitamin-c-and-cancer.

28   E. Cameron and L. Pauling, "Supplemental ascorbate in the supportive treatment of cancer: Prolongation of survival times in terminal human cancer," Proceedings of the National Academy of Sciences of the United States of America, October 1976, 73(10):3685-9;

29   A. Murata and F. Morishige, International Conference on Nutrition, Taijin, China 1981. Report in Medical Tribune (22/6/81) A. Murata, et al, "Prolongation of survival times of terminal cancer patients by administration of large doses of ascorbate," International Journal for Vitamin and Nutrition Research, Suppl, 1982;23:103-13

30   E.T. Creagan, et al, "Failure of high-dose vitamin C (ascorbic acid) therapy to benefit patients with advanced cancer. A controlled trial," *New England Journal of Medicine*, September 27, 1979, 301(13):687-90

31   MA Moyad, MA Combs, AS Vrablic, J Velasquez, B Turner, and S Bernal, "Vitamin C metabolites, independent of smoking status, significantly enhance leukocyte, but not plasma ascorbate concentrations," *Advances in Therapy* 2008; 25: 995-1009.

32   CS Johnston and B Luo, "Comparison of the absorption and excretion of three commercially available sources of vitamin C," *Journal of the American Dietetic Association* 1994;94:779-81

33   Institute of Medicine. Food and Nutrition Board. Dietary Reference Intakes for Vitamin C, Vitamin E, Selenium, and Carotenoids. (Washington, DC: National Academy Press, 2000).

34   *The Whole Foods Encyclopedia*. (New York: Prentice-Hall, 1988). PMID: 15220.

35 "Can Tumeric reduce the spread of Breast Cancer," American College for Advancement in Medicine, Integrative Medicine Blog, March 10, 2010, http://www.acam.org/blogpost/1092863/ACAM-Integrative-Medicine-Blog?tag=tumeric.

36 Aggarwal B. Paper presented at the U.S. Defense Department's "Era of Hope" Breast Cancer Research Program meeting in Philadelphia, PA, October 5, 2005, reported in NUTRAingredients.com/Europe

37 "Turmeric slows breast cancer spread in mice," Constitutive NF-kappaB activation, induces G1/S arrest, suppresses proliferation, and induces apoptosis in mantle cell lymphoma. Biochem Pharmacol. September 1, 2005, 70(5):700-13. 2005. PMID:16023083.

38 RF Tayyem, DD Heath, WK Al-Delaimy, and CL Rock, "Curcumin content of turmeric and curry powders," *Nutr Cancer.* 2006;55(2):126-31. 2006. PMID:17044766

39 S Shapiro, R Farmer, J Stevenson, H Burger, and A Mueck, "Does Hormone Replacement Therapy Cause Breast Cancer?" *Journal of Family Planning and Reproductive Health Care,* 2012;38(2):102-109. © 2012

40 http://www.webmd.com/menopause/features/hrt-revisiting-the-hormone-decision

41 J. Mercola, "Hormone Replacement Therapy," May 8, 2013, http://articles.mercola.com/sites/articles/archive/2013/08/05/hormone-replacement-therapy.aspx

Chapter 5

1 C DeSantis, S Fedewa, A.G. Sauer, J Kramer, R Smith, and A Jernal, Breast Cancer Statistics, 2015:Convergence of Incidence Rates between Black and White Women, CA Cancer J Clin 2016; 66:31-42.

2 J Fernandez-Cornejo, S Wechsler, M Livingston, and L Mitchell, "Genetically Engineered Crops in the United States," February 2014, http://www.ers.usda.gov/media/1282246/err162.pdf.

3 http://www.aaemonline.org/gmopost.html

4 B Stoffel, "10 Foods You'll Have to Give Up to Avoid Eating GMOs," November 21, 203, http://www.dailyfinance.com/2013/11/21/foods-give-up-avoid-eating-gmo/.

5 C Tjol, "The unspoken link between GM-foods and cancer," September 15, 2014, http://www.naturalnews.com/046742_GMOs_cancer_Monsanto.html.

6   R Klement and U Kammerer, "Is there a role for carbohydrate restriction in the treatment and prevention of cancer?" *Nutrition & Metabolism* 2011, 8:75 http://www.nutritionandmetabolism.com/content/8/1/75.

7   M Marchione, "Eating Lots of Carbs May Raise the Risk of Breast Cancer, Study Shows," AP, 2011, http://jonnybowden.com/high-carb-diets-and-breast-cancer-risk/.

8   JY Dong and LQ Qin, "Dietary glycemic index, glycemic load, and risk of breast cancer: meta- analysis of prospective cohort studies," Breast Cancer Res Treat 2011; 126: 287–94.

9   http://www.diabetes.org/food-and-fitness/food/what-can-i-eat/understanding-carbohydrates/glycemic-index-and-diabetes.html

10   http://www.medindia.net/patients/calculators/glycemic-index.asp

11   http://naldc.nal.usda.gov/naldc/download.xhtml?id=CAT10842840&content=PDF

12   A Curry, "Archaeology: The milk revolution," *Nature International Weekly Journal of Science*, July 31, 2013, from http://www.nature.com/news/archaeology-the-milk-revolution-1.13471.

13   http://drbenkim.com/articles-dairy.html

14   Peter D'Adamo and Catherine Whitney. *Eat Right 4 (for) Your Type: The Individualized Diet Solution to Staying Healthy, Living Longer & Achieving Your Ideal Weight: 4 Blood Types, 4 Diets*, (New York: G.P. Putnam's Sons, 1996).

15   C Kroenke, M Kwan, C Sweeney, A Castillo, and B Caan, "High and Low Fat Dairy Intake, Recurrence, and Mortality after Breast Cancer Diagnosis," *Journal of the National Cancer Institute*, April 30, 2013 http://jnci.oxfordjournals.org/content/early/2013/03/08/jnci.djt027.abstract.

16   http://www.breastcancer.org/research-news/20130327

17   C Hicks, "Give Up Dairy Products to Beat Cancer," *The Telegraph*, June 2, 2014, http://www.telegraph.co.uk/foodanddrink/healthyeating/10868428/Give-up-dairy-products-to- beat-cancer.html.

18   "Seventh Day Adventist Diet" http://www.nutrition411.com/articles/seventh-day-adventist-diet-0

19   http://www.pcrm.org/health/cancer-resources/diet-cancer/facts/meat-consumption-and-cancer- risk

20   World Cancer Research Fund. "Food, nutrition, physical activity, and the prevention of cancer: A global perspective." American Institute of Cancer Research. Washington, DC: 2007.

21   International Agency for Cancer Research, World Health Organization, October 26, 2015, http://www.iarc.fr/en/media-centre/pr/2015/pdfs/pr240_E.) pdf

22   TJ Key, PN Appleby, EA Spencer, et al, "Cancer incidence in British vegetarians," *British Journal of Cancer.* 2009; 101:192–197

23   www.vibrantlife.com

24   J. Mercola, "Glyphosate drives breast cancer proliferation, study warns, as urine tests show Europeans have this weed killer in their body," June 25, 2013, http://articles.mercola.com/sites/articles/archive/2013/06/25/glyphosate-residue.aspx.

25   Kaayla Daniel, *The Whole Soy Story: The Dark Side of America's Favorite Health Food*, (New Trends Publishing, 2005).

26   http://www.natural-health-cafe.org/macrobiotic-eating.html#.Vy8cY4-cGUk

27   Bob Arnot, *The Breast Cancer Prevention Diet*, (Little, Brown and Company, 1998).

28   Advanced Nutrition Publications, Inc. Nutritional Influences on Estrogen Metabolism. Applied Nutritional Science Reports, Met451, 2001

29   Calcium-D-glucarate. Altern Med Rev. Aug; 7(4);336-9.

30   http://wikiwel.com/wikihealing//index.php?title=Diindolylmethane

31   http://www.wellnessresources.com/health/articles/i3c_and_dim_for_breast_prostate_cancer_prevention/

32   B Richards, "I3C and DIM for Breast & Prostate Cancer Prevention," October 11, 2012, http://www.wellnessresources.com/health/articles/i3c_and_dim_for_breast_prostate_cancer_prevention/.

33   R. Webster Kehr, "High-Dose Intravenous Vitamin C (IVC)," Independent Cancer Research Foundation, Inc, March 1, 2015, http://www.cancertutor.com/vitaminc_ivc/.

34   G. Block, "Epidemiologic evidence regarding vitamin C and cancer," *American Journal of Clinical Nutrition.* 1991 Dec;54(6 Suppl):1310S-1314S. http://www.ncbi.nlm.nih.gov/pubmed/1962588.

35   Gandini, *European Journal of Cancer* (2000);36:636-46.

36   https://www.nlm.nih.gov/medlineplus/ency/article/002404.htm

37   http://whfoods.org/genpage.php?tname=nutrient&dbid=109&utm_source=feedly_reader&utm_medium=rss&utm_campaign=rss_feed

38   Riordan Clinic. Seasonal Defense: Boosting Your Immune System. https://riordanclinic.org/2011/11/seasonal-defense-boosting-your-immune-system/

39   US Department of Agriculture, Agricultural Research Service. 2011. USDA National Nutrient Database for Standard Reference, Release 24. Nutrient Data Laboratory Home Page, http://www.ars.usda.gov/ba/bhnrc/ndl.

40   Tim O'Shea, "Natural Whole Food Vitamins: Ascorbic Acid is Not Vitamin C," 2009 http://www.thedoctorwithin.com/vitaminc/ascorbic-acid-is-not-vitamin-c/.

41   Mark Levine, et al, "Determination of optimal vitamin C requirements in humans," *American Journal of Clinical Nutrition*, Vol. 62, 1995, pp. 1347S-56S.

42   Mark Levine, et al, "Vitamin C pharmacokinetics in healthy volunteers: Evidence for a recommended dietary allowance." Proceedings of the National Academy of Sciences USA, Vol. 93, No. 8, April 16, 1996, pp. 3704-09.

43   https://www.consumerlab.com/reviews/vitamin-C_supplement_review/vitaminc/

44   AS Prasad, FW Beck, DC Snell, and O Kucuk, "Zinc in Cancer Prevention." *Nutr Cancer*, 2009;61(6):879-87. doi: 10.1080/01635580903285122. http://www.ncbi.nlm.nih.gov/pubmed/20155630.

45   B.N. Ames and P. Wakimoto, "Are vitamin and mineral deficiencies a major cancer risk?" *Nat. Rev. Cancer* 2002, 2, 694-704.

46   Institute of Medicine, Food and Nutrition Board. Dietary Reference Intakes for Vitamin A, Vitamin K, Arsenic, Boron, Chromium, Copper, Iodine, Iron, Manganese, Molybdenum, Nickel, Silicon, Vanadium, and Zinc. Washington, DC: National Academy Press, 2001.

47   AS Prasad, "Zinc: an overview," *Nutrition* 1995;11:93-9.

48   US Department of Agriculture, Agricultural Research Service. 2011. USDA National Nutrient Database for Standard Reference, Release 24. Nutrient Data Laboratory Home Page, http://www.ars.usda.gov/ba/bhnrc/ndl.

49   http://naturalsociety.com/two-must-minerals-fighting-breast-cancer/

50   D.K. Dhawan and Vijayta D. Chadha, "Zinc: A promising agent in dietary chemoprevention of cancer," *Indian Journal of Medical Research*, 2010 Dec; 132(6): 676–682.http://www.ncbi.nlm.nih.gov/pmc/articles/PMC3102454/.

51   AS Prasad, FW Beck, DC Snell, and O Kucuk, "Zinc in Cancer Prevention," *Nutrition and Cancer*, 2009;61(6):879-87. doi: 10.1080/01635580903285122. http://www.ncbi.nlm.nih.gov/pubmed/20155630.

52 Barbara L. Minton. "Zinc and Selenium are the Minerals that Fight Breast Cancer," May 24, 2009, http://www.naturalnews.com/026321_zinc_cancer_selenium.html.

53 Group E., 7 Common Types of Zinc Explained. Global Health Center. December 11, 2009. http://www.globalhealingcenter.com/natural-health/types-of-zinc/

54 Kayla Grossmann. "Are you Zinc Deficient? A simple DIY test from Premier Research Labs," 2014 .http://blog.radiantlifecatalog.com/bid/59012/Are-you-Zinc-Deficient-A-simple-DIY- test-from-Premier-Research-Labs

55 RA Sunde, Selenium. In: Ross AC, Caballero B, Cousins RJ, Tucker KL, Ziegler TR, eds. Modern Nutrition in Health and Disease. 11th ed. Philadelphia, PA: Lippincott Williams & Wilkins; 2012:225-37

56 http://www.whfoods.com/genpage.php?dbid=95&tname=nutrient

57 M Loef, GN Schrauzer, and H Walach, "Selenium and Alzheimer's disease: a systematic review," J Alzheimers Dis 2011;26:81-104.

58 S Suzanna, BG Cham, G Ahmad Rohi, R Mohd Rizal, MN Fairulnizal, H Normah, and A Fatimah, "Relationship between selenium and breast cancer: a case-control study in the Klang Valley," Singapore Medical Journal, March 2009, 50(3):265-9. http://www.ncbi.nlm.nih.gov/pubmed/19352569.

59 RA Sunde, Selenium. In: Ross AC, Caballero B, Cousins RJ, Tucker KL, Ziegler TR, eds. Modern Nutrition in Health and Disease. 11th ed. Philadelphia, PA: Lippincott Williams & Wilkins; 2012:225-37.

60 SB Goldhaber, "Trace element risk assessment: essentiality vs toxicity," Regul Toxicol Pharmacol. 2003 Oct;38(2):232-42. http://www.ncbi.nlm.nih.gov/pubmed/14550763

61 http://www.greenmedinfo.com/blog/confirmed-flaxseed-contains-estrogens-regress-cancer

62 http://www.klactive.com/metaflax/

63 http://fitlifeofcolorado.com/Resources/ID/81/The-Benefits-of-Flaxseed

64 H Adlercreutz, "Lignans and Human Health," Critical Reviews in Clinical Laboratory Science. 2007;44(5-6):483-525. http://www.ncbi.nlm.nih.gov/pubmed/17943494.

65 J Nordqvist, "Flaxseed: Health Benefits, Facts, Research," Medical News Today, January 11, 2016, http://www.medicalnewstoday.com/articles/263405.php?page=2.

66 LU Thompson, JM Chen, T Li, K Strasser-Weippl, and PE Goss, "Dietary flaxseed alters tumor biological markers in postmenopausal

breast cancer," Clin Cancer Res. 2005 May 15; 11(10):3828-35 from http://www.ncbi.nlm.nih.gov/pubmed/15897583.

67   http://umm.edu/health/medical/altmed/herb/flaxseed

68   Mabel M. Esten and Albert G. Dannin, (1950) "Chlorophyll therapy and its relation to pathogenic bacteria." Butler University Botanical Studies : Vol. 9, Article 21.

69   C Jubert, J Mata, G Bench, R Dashwood, C Pereira, W Tracewell, K Turteltaub, D Williams, and G Bailey, "Effects of chlorophyll and chlorophyllin on low-dose aflatoxin B(1) pharmacokinetics in human volunteers," *Cancer Prevention Research* (Phila). 2009 Dec;2

70   YL Zhang, L Guan, PH Zhou, LJ Mao, ZM Zhao, SQ Li, XX Xu, CC Cong, MX Zhu, and JY Zhao, "The protective effect of chlorophyllin against oxidative damage and its mechanism," Zhonghua Nei Ke Za Zhi. 2012 Jun;51(6):466-70

71   http://superhealthsupplements.com/chlorophyll-ageing/

72   http://hippocratesinst.org/benefits-of-wheatgrass-2

73   http://www.tellmymom.com/22-239.html

74   http://umm.edu/health/medical/altmed/supplement/omega6-fatty-acids

75   http://www.suma.coop/resources/information-sheets/essential-fatty-acids/

76   U. Nair and H. Bartsch, "Lipid peroxidation-induced DNA damage in cancer-prone inflammatory diseases: a review of published adduct types and levels in humans." *Free Radical Biology & Medicine*, October 15, 2007, 43(8):1109-20 Epub July 20, 2007, http://www.ncbi.nlm.nih.gov/pubmed/17854706.

77   http://ww5.komen.org/BreastCancer/LowerYourRiskReferences.html

78   S Sieri, et al, "Consuming a high-fat diet is associated with increased risk of certain types of BC," *Journal of the National Cancer Institute.* April 9, 2014, http://jnci.oxfordjournals.org/content/early/2014/04/04/jnci.dju114.full.

79   S. Simon, "How Your Weight Affects Your Risk of Breast Cancer," October 13, 2014, http://www.cancer.org/cancer/news/features/how-your-weight-affects-your-risk-of-breast-cancer.

80   http://www.healthy.net/Health/Essay/Breast_Health_Tip_21_Avoid_Sugar/696

81   Robert H. Lustig, Laura A. Schmidt, and Claire D. Brindis, "The Toxic Truth about Sugar." *Nature* 482 (2012): 27-29.

82   C Duchaine, I Dumas, and C Diorio, "Comsumption of sweet foods and mammographic breast density: A cross-sectional study," *BioMed Central*

Public Health. 2014; 14 ;554 http://www.ncbi.nlm.nih.gov/pmc/articles/PMC4071328/.

83   http://www.bengaloncology.org/cancer_sugar_facts.html

84   http://www.newliving.com/issues/aug-2005/articles/breast%20cancer.html

85   M Soffritti, F Belpoggi, DD Esposti, L Lambertini, E Tibaldi, and A Rigano, DOI,10.1289/ehp.8711. Online November 17, 2005.

86   World Health Organization website. "Global Status report on alcohol and health," World Health Organization, 2014. http://www.who.int/substance_abuse/publications/global_alcohol_report/msbgsruprofiles.pdf

87   A Mordey, "Does Alcohol Cause Breast Cancer," The Cabin Chiang Mai. May 19, 2014, http://www.thecabinchiangmai.com/blog/does_alcohol_cause_breast_cancer_#.Vq55hY-cGUk.

88   T. Key, P. Appleby, I Barnes, and G. Reeves, "Endogenous sex hormones and breast cancer in postmenopausal women: reanalysis of nine prospective studies. *Journal of the National Cancer Institute*, 2002, 94, 606-16. Accessed February 24, 2016.

89   M.A. Korsten, "Alcoholism and pancreatitis: Does nutrition play a role?" *Alcohol Health & Research World* 13(3):232-237, 1989.

90   http://www.cancer.gov/about-cancer/causes-prevention/risk/alcohol/alcohol-fact-sheet

91   "Million Women Study Shows Even Moderate Alcohol consumption Associated with Increased Cancer Risk," *Journal of the National Cancer Institute*, V101, (5)p281 http://jnci.oxfordjournals.org/content/101/5/281.2.full.

92   http://www.healthyeatingadvisor.com/9cancer-causingchemicals.html

93   Copyright © Environmental Working Group,www.ewg.org. http://www.ewg.org/research/ewg-s-dirty-dozen-guide-food-additives

94   L.B. Dusdieker, et al, "Nitrate in baby foods. Adding to the nitrate mosaic." *Arch. Pediatr. Adolesc. Med.*, 1994 148(5):490-494.

95   https://www.epa.gov/sites/production/files/2015-04/documents/nitrate_0.pdf

96   *Journal of Applied Toxicology* March 2012; 32(3): 219-232

97   https://ntp.niehs.nih.gov/ntp/roc/content/profiles/butylatedhydroxyanisole.pdf

98   http://oehha.ca.gov/chemicals/butylated-hydroxyanisole

99   M Maffini, "Losing our minds: the ongoing chemicals' attack on our children's brains," National Resources Defense council Staff

Blog, May 29, 2014 http://switchboard.nrdc.org/blogs/mmaffini/losing_our_minds_the_ongoing_c.html

100 Ter Veld et al, "Scientific Opinion on the re-evaluation of Propyl Gallate (E310) as a food additive," April 24, 2014; EFSA Journal 2014;12(4):3642 [46 pp.].

101 William Marias Malisoff (1943), *Dictionary of Bio-Chemistry and Related Subjects*, Philosophical Library. pp. 311, 530, 573.

102 https://en.wikipedia.org/wiki/Theobromine

103 http://www.ncbi.nlm.nih.gov/pubmed/8280834

104 http://www.ewg.org/research/ewg-s-dirty-dozen-guide-food-additives/fda-failed-us

105 A. Downham and P. Collins, "Colouring our foods in the last and next millennium," *International Journal of Food Science and Technology*, December 25, 2001, DOI: 10.1046/j.1365-2621.2000.00373.x from http://onlinelibrary.wiley.com/doi/10.1046/j.1365-2621.2000.00373.x/abstract;jsessionid=C9726B66FCEA6ED2761420654537617F.f03t02

106 http://www.wholefoodsmagazine.com/news/breaking-news/artificial-food-dyes-can-cause- cancer-adhd

107 http://www.healthyeatingadvisor.com/9cancer-causingchemicals.html

108 R. Rutledge, "Gasping for Action," *Journal Sentinel*, February 14, 2015, http://www.jsonline.com/watchdog/watchdogreports/gasping-for-action-b99440601z1-291548941.html

109 http://www.nbcnews.com/id/20605135/ns/health-health_care/t/major-popcorn-makers-drop- toxic-chemical/#.VeTxMjZRGUk

110 C. Potera, "Diet and Nutrition: Phosphate linked to lung cancer in mice," *Environmental Health Perspectives*, March 2009 http://www.ncbi.nlm.nih.gov/pmc/articles/PMC2661925/ Reproduced with permission from Environmental Health Perspectives http://www.ncbi.nlm.nih.gov/pmc/articles/PMC2661925/

111 H. Hafer, "The Hidden Drug Dietary Phosphate," http://www.phosadd.com/foods/foodselection.htm.

112 C. Exley, LM Charles, L. Barr, C. Martin, A. Polwart, and P.D. Darbre, "Aluminum in human breast tissue," J Inorg Biochem. September 2007, 101(9):1344-6. Epub June 12, 2007. http://www.ncbi.nlm.nih.gov/pubmed/17629949/.

113 E Helsing, "Traditional diets and disease patterns of the Mediterranean, circa 1960," *The American Society for Clinical Nutrition*, 1995. http://ajcn.nutrition.org/content/61/6/1329S.abstract.

114 http://www.nutrition-and-you.com/purslane.html

115 http://www.wcrf.org/int/cancer-facts-figures/data-specific-cancers/ breast-cancer-statistics

116 D Larsen, "The 5 Places Where People Live the Longest," Senior Living Blog, July 21, 2014, http://www.aplaceformom.com/ blog/2013-03-29-where-people-live-the-longest/.

117 "Circulating Carotenoids and Risk of breast cancer: Pooled Analysis of Eight Prospective Studies," *Journal of the National Cancer Institute*, December 18, 2012, http://jnci.oxfordjournals.org/content/early/2012/12/05/jnci. djs461.abstract?sid=a11a72f8-1cb5-4c39-9a90-722cbbd0d5ab.

118 https://www.veganmainstream.com/2013/06/28/feature-interview- dr-pam-popper-on-her-new- book-food-over-medicine/

119 J Mercola, "Why Food Addictions can be as Strong as Drug Addictions," July 13, 2011, from http://articles.mercola.com/sites/articles/ archive/2011/07/13/why-food-addictions-can-be-as-strong-as-drug- addictions.aspx.

Chapter 6

1 Dr. Henry Mallek. *The New Longevity Diet*. (The Berkley Publishing Group, 2001). 54-80, 107-119.

2 http://www.letstalkconstipation.com/living/

3 Hye-Rim Lee, Kyung-A Hwang, Ki-Hoan Nam, Hyoung-Chin Kim, and Kyung-Chul, ***Chio***. *Chemical Research in Toxicology*., 2014, *27* (5), pp 834–842.Publication Date (Web): March 31, 2014 Copyright © 2014 American Chemical Society. http://pubs.acs.org/doi/abs/10.1021/ tx5000156. Progression of Breast Cancer Cells Was Enhanced by Endocrine-Disrupting Chemicals, Triclosan and Octylphenol

4 www.Dollstatus.com

Chapter 7

1 KY Wolin, K Carson, and GA Colditz, "Obesity and cancer," *Oncologist* 2010; 15(6):556–565

2 http://www.asco.org/practice-research/obesity-and-cancer

3 http://www.cancer.gov/about-cancer/causes-prevention/risk/obesity/ obesity-fact-sheet

4 http://jama.jamanetwork.com/article.aspx?articleid=1832542

5 http://www.nhlbi.nih.gov/health/educational/lose_wt/bmitools.htm

6 http://www.nhlbi.nih.gov/health/educational/lose_wt/BMI/ bmicalc.htm

7   http://www.niddk.nih.gov/health-information/health-statistics/Pages/overweight-obesity-statistics.aspx

8   http://www.msgtruth.org/whatisit.htm

9   http://www.foodsafey.gov/FDA and Monosodium glutamate (MSG), August 31, 1995

10   J. Mercola, "MSG: Is this Silent Killer Lurking in Your Kitchen Cabinets," April 21, 2009, http://articles.mercola.com/sites/articles/archive/2009/04/21/msg-is-this-silent-killer-lurking-in-your-kitchen-cabinets.aspx

11   ND Volkow, et al, "'Nonhedonic' food motivation in humans involves dopamine in the dorsal striatum and methylphenidate amplifies this effect," *Synapse*, June 1, 2002, 44(3):175-80. http://www.ncbi.nlm.nih.gov/pubmed/11954049#openModal.

12   Nicole M. Avena, Pedro Rada, and Bartley G. Hoebel, "Evidence for sugar addiction: Behavioral and neurochemical effects of intermittent, excessive sugar intake," *Neuroscience & Biobehavioral Reviews*, 2008; 32(1): 20–39. http://www.ncbi.nlm.nih.gov/pmc/articles/PMC2235907/

13   M. Hyman, *The Blood Sugar Solution: The ultrahealthy program for losing weight, preventing disease, and feeling great now!* (New York: Little, Brown and Co., 2012).

14   M. Hyman, "Food Addiction: Could it explain why 70 percent of America is fat," October 18, 2014, http://drhyman.com/blog/2011/02/04/food-addiction-could-it-explain-why-70-percent-of-america-is-fat/#close.

15   http://www.webmd.com/diet/features/emotional-eating-feeding-your-feelings

16   July 2000, American Demographics from https://www.researchgate.net/journal/0163-4089_American_demographics

17   P.J. D'Adamo and C. Whitney, *Eat Right for Your Type*, (New York: G.P. Putnam's Sons, 1996).

18   I. Lee, et al, "Effect of physical inactivity on major non-communicable diseases worldwide: an analysis of burden of disease and life expectancy," Lancet, 2012. 380: p. 219-29.

19   http://www.ginapersonaltraining.co.uk/benefits-of-fitness/

20   https://www.fredhutch.org/en/events/healthy-living/Trim-Risk.html

21   National Center for Chronic Disease Prevention and Health Promotion and Centers for Disease Control and Prevention (1996). *Physical Activity and Health: A Report of the Surgeon General*. Retrieved June 26, 2009, from http://www.cdc.gov/nccdphp/sgr/pdf/execsumm.pdf

22 TM Peters, SC Moore, GL Gierach, NJ Wareham, U Ekelund, AR Hollenbeck, A Schatzkin, and MF Leitzmann, "Intensity and timing of physical activity in relation to postmenopausal breast cancer risk: the prospective NIH-AARP diet and health study," BMC Cancer 9 (2009) 349. doi:10.1186/1471-2407-9-349

23 P Bonanno, "Study Shows Exercise Lowers Cancer and Recurrence," September 4, 2014, http://nwhc.net/blog/study-shows-exercise-lowers-risk-of-breast-cancer-and-recurrence.

24 http://www.aacr.org/Newsroom/Pages/News-Release-Detail.aspx?ItemID=580#.VTb1THJFCUk

25 http://www.everydayhealth.com/fitness/workouts/tips/calculate-your-target-heart-rate.aspx

26 Cancer Epidemiol Biomarkers Prev December 2012 21:2209-2219; Published Online First October 16, 2012; doi:10.1158/1055-9965.EPI-12-0961

27 M. Allen, "Cycling Training Tips: Cycling helps beat cancer," April 30, 2010, http://www.bicycling.com/training/fitness/cycling-training-tips-cycling-helps-beat-cancer.

Chapter 8

1 http://besynchro.com/blogs/blog/12492461-xenoestrogens-plastics-dirty-secret

2 A Samsel and S Seneff, "Glyphosate, pathways to modern diseases II: Celiac sprue and gluten intolerance," *Interdisciplinary Toxicology*, December 2013, 6(4): 159–184 http://www.ncbi.nlm.nih.gov/pmc/articles/PMC3945755/.

3 http://people.howstuffworks.com/epa3.htm

4 https://en.wikipedia.org/wiki/Endocrine_disruptor

5 "Dirty dozen endocrine disruptors," October 28, 2013, http://www.ewg.org/research/dirty- dozen-list-endocrine-disruptors*.

6 http://www.niehs.nih.gov/health/topics/agents/sya-bpa/

7 J Rochester, A Bolden, and "Bishenol S and F: A Systematic review and comparison of the hormonal activity of bisphenol A substitutes," *Environmental Health Perspectives*, DOI:10.1289/ehp.1408989, http://ehp.niehs.nih.gov/1408989/

8 http://www.ejnet.org/dioxin/.

9 M Warner, B Eskenazi, P Mocarelli, P Gerthoux, S Samuals, L Needham, D Patterson, and P Brambilla, "Serum dioxin concentrations and breast cancer risk in the Seveso women's health study," *Environmental Health*

Perspectives, July 2002, 110(7): 625–628 http://www.ncbi.nlm.nih.gov/pmc/articles/PMC1240906/.

[10] A Schecter, P Cramer, K Boggess, J Stanley, O Papke, J Olson, A Silver, and M Schmitz, "Intake of Dioxins and related compounds from food in the U.S. population," *Journal of Toxicology and Environmental Health*, Part A, 63:1-18, 2001 http://www.ejnet.org/dioxin/dioxininfood.pdf.

[11] http://www.savethefrogs.com/threats/pesticides/atrazine/index.html

[12] http://ehp.niehs.nih.gov/0901091/

[13] F Chen and M Chien, "Lower concentrations of phthalates induce proliferation in human breast cancer cells," *Climacteric* Vol 17, Issue 4, 2014 http://www.tandfonline.com/doi/abs/10.3109/13697137.2013.865720?journalCode=icmt20#.VdpZeI5RHX4.

[14] "Research calls for use of molecular iodine to treat breast cancer," *Market Wire*, October 2006, http://findarticles.com/p/articles/mi_pwwi/is_200610/ai_n16809836/.

[15] http://www.hbo.com/documentaries/toxic-hot-seat/synopsis.html

[16] OI Alatise and GN Schrauzer, "Lead exposure: A contributing cause of the current breast cancer epidemic in Nigerian women," *Biological Trace Element Research*, August 2010, 13 6(2):127-39. doi: 10.1007/s12011-010-8608-2. Epub March 3, 2010, http://www.ncbi.nlm.nih.gov/pubmed/20195925.

[17] C Siewit, B Gengler, E Vegas, R Puckett, and M Louie, "Cadmium promotes breast cancer cell proliferation by potentiating the interaction between ERα and c-Jun," *Molecular Endocrinology*, May 2010.24(5): 981–992, Published online March 10, 2010, doi: 10.1210/me.2009-0410 from http://www.ncbi.nlm.nih.gov/pmc/articles/PMC2870938/.

[18] http://pennstatehershey.adam.com/content.aspx?productId=117&pid=1&gid=002473

[19] A Smith, G Marshall, Y Yuan, C Steinmaus, J Liaw, M Smith, L Wood, M Meirich, R Fritzemeier, M Pegram, and C Ferreccio, "Rapid Reduction in Breast Cancer Mortality with Inorganic Arsenic in Drinking Water," eBioMed Vol(1) Issue 1, P 58-63, November 2014 http://www.sciencedirect.com/science/article/pii/S2352396414000073.

[20] http://healthywildandfree.com/4-ways-people-are-increasing-their-childs-cancer-risk/

[21] http://www.nrdc.org/health/effects/mercury/guide.asp

[22] V. Stejskal, A. Danersud, A. Lindvall, R. Hudecek, V. Nordman, A. Yaqob, W. Mayer, W. Bieger, and U. Lindh, "Metal-Specific Memory

Lymphocytes; Biomarkers of Sensitivity in Man," Neuroendocrinology Letters 1999; 20: 221-289

23   P. Darbre, A. Aljarrah, and W. Miller, 2004, "Concentrations of parabens in human breast tumours," *Journal of Applied Toxicologyl*, 24, 5–13.

24   http://coeh.berkeley.edu/greenchemistry/cbcrp.htm

25   http://www.nomorebreastcancer.org.uk/common_carcinogens.html

26   http://www.atsdr.cdc.gov/substances/toxsubstance.asp?toxid=16

27   http://www.healthychild.org/easy-steps/avoid-alkylphenol-ethoxylates-apes-in-cleaning- products-and-more/

28   http://www.safecosmetics.org/get-the-facts/chemicals-of-concern/

Chapter 9

1   http://www.miracleessentialoils.com/howto/index.php?subid=G-top-usingessentialoils&gclid=CPClkc_su8sCFQeraQodTyACTQ

2   Aroma Tools Modern Essentials App. for Android. 2016

Chapter 10

1   *Journal of Personality and Social Psychology.* June 1998, 74(6):1646-55, http://www.ncbi.nlm.nih.gov/pubmed/9654763.

2   Caroline Myss, *Why People Don't Heal.* (Three Rivers Press is a trademark of Random House, 1997) 25.

3   Emotions and Health, NIH Medline Plus: the magazine [Internet]. 2008 Winter [cited 2016 January 16]; 3(1): 4 available from http://www.nlm.nih.gov/medlineplus/magazine/issues/winter08/articles/winter08pg4.html.

4   F Mancini, "Are You Half-full or Half empty?" http://drfabmancini.com/blog/

6   Wayne W. Dyer, *Your Sacred Self,* (Harper Collins Publishers, 1995) 298.

7   S Pavlina, "How to Discover your Life Purpose in About 20 Minutes," Podcast, 7.21.2011 http://www.learnoutloud.com/podcasts/PGP-072111.mp3.

8   www.stress.org/stress-effects

9   Copyright © 2014 HeartMath LLC. All Rights Reserved. http://www.heartmath.com/infographics/how-stress-affects-the-body/.

10   M Moreno-Smith, SK Lutgendorf, and AK Sood, "Impact of stress on cancer metastasis," *Future Oncology*, 2010;6(12):1863-1881.

11   A Scholberg, "The doctor who cured too many patients," http://www.cancerdefeated.com/newsletters/The-doctor-who-cured%20too-many-patients.html.

12   http://www.nlm.nih.gov/medlineplus/magazine/issues/winter08/articles/winter08pg4.html

13   L Nummenmaa, E Glerean, R Hari, and J Hietanen, "Bodily maps of emotions," Proceedings of the National Academy of Sciences, vol. 111 no. 2, Lauri Nummenmaa, 646–651, doi: 10.1073/pnas.1321664111 from http://www.pnas.org/content/111/2/646.abstract?tab=author-info.

14   "The Making of Emotions," May 30, 2015, https://www.heartmath.org/articles-of-the- heart/science-of-the-heart/making-emotions/.

15   Stephen R. Covey, *The 7 Habits of Highly Effective People: Restoring the Character Ethic.* [Rev. ed.]. (New York: Free Press, 2004).

Let's Wrap It Up

1   http://www.breastcancer.org/symptoms/understand_bc/statistics

2   J. Gofman, 1999, Radiation from Medical Procedures in the Pathogenesis of Cancer and Ischemic Heart Disease: Dose-response Studies with Physicians per 100,000 Population. San Francisco: CNR Book Division, Committee for Nuclear Responsibility.

3   G. Heyes, A. Mill, and M. Charles, 2009, Mammography: oncogenecity at low doses. J Radiol Protect, 29, 123–132.

Made in the USA
Monee, IL
02 January 2022

87757489R00142